First Aid Dentistry

An Illustrated History of Dental Practice by a U.S. Army Surgeon – Tooth Extraction, Diseases of the Mouth, Fractures of the Jaw and Operative Procedures

By Edward P. R. Ryan

First Lieutenant and Dental Surgeon, United States Army

With 80 Illustrations

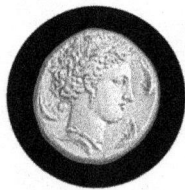

PANTIANOS
CLASSICS

Published by Pantianos Classics

ISBN-13: 978-1-78987-126-5

First published in 1914

Contents

Disclaimer

The contents of this book depict dental procedures and treatments of the early 20th century. The information herein is presented for entertainment and historical purposes only. By reading this text, the reader assumes all responsibility for any negative consequences or harm resulting from the improper use of the material presented.

Preface

This book has been designed for medical and dental practitioners and students, for nurses; and especially for hospital corps men of the military and naval service and for all who are called upon to administer relief from dental pain, where the services of a dental surgeon cannot be obtained.

The impulse prompting this book was not to multiply books, but arose from the writer's belief and that expressed by many practitioners, both medical and dental, that this hand-book is needed by those it is intended to serve.

The extent and scope of the methods described are limited to **First Aid,** which will relieve the patient from suffering until a dental surgeon may complete the treatment. A minimum number of instruments is recommended and their use shown and described.

The methods used are simple and the descriptions have been written in the simplest words, technical terms being eliminated as much as possible; all methods used can be accomplished on board ship or in the field or in any hospital or medical office.

Due credit is given the works of modern writers, which have been consulted and without them it would have been impossible to accomplish what has been done.

The gratitude of the writer is here expressed to Captain J. R. Harris, M. C, U. S. Army, for valuable suggestions and assistance; and special credit is due Mr. H. A. Utter for photos from which these illustrations were made.

The Author.

Chapter One - Septic Conditions of the Mouth

The writer does not intend to go out of his sphere and make suggestions as to the treatment and diagnosis of disease in general, but merely to present some ideas from a dental standpoint which, in their connection with systemic conditions, are frequently overlooked.

In the present-day importance of opsonia and vaccine therapy and the treatment of diseased conditions by these methods, greater emphasis should be placed on the condition of the mouth, with regard to the presence of pathogenic bacteria. The oral cavity is an ideal location for the cultivation of bacteria. Nutrient material is abundant, as well as a proper temperature and in most mouths, predisposition.

Consider a mouth containing many necrosed roots, at times floating in pus; teeth covered by tartar, crowding the tissue and preserving undisturbed shelves under the margins of the gums, for retention of decomposing food matter; cavities full of foul germ-laden substance; ill-fitting crowns, plates and fillings. It is hard to imagine more favorable conditions than these for the growth of. disease-producing germs.

Miller [1] found upward of one hundred organisms in the mouth, thirteen varieties being common, with the following pus-producing organisms:

Staphylococcus pyogenes aureus..........................34.8% of cases.
Streptococcus. Pyogenes.....................................23.2% of cases.
Staphylococcus pyogenes albus............................18.6% of cases.
Bacillus pyocyaneus...9.3 % of cases.
Staphylococcus pyogenes citrus..........................4.6% of cases.

The other eight varieties being harmless and varying in frequency. The fact that the staphylococcus and streptococcus organisms, the most active of pathogenic germs, are present to this enormous extent, should impress upon us the importance of the mouth as an etiological factor in disease.

The presence of these organisms is not to be considered merely as a cause of inflammation, stomatitis, gingivitis and local effects, which are seen; but it must be further considered that the mucous membrane of the rest of the alimentary tract has probably less power of resistance than the mouth. The wonderful resisting power which the mucosa of the oral cavity exerts and its ability to rebuild after injury is known to all, but this power is exerted only to resist for itself and to throw off, not to destroy or render less infectious, the cultures we swallow continually.

The presence of pyorrhea is not the only cause of many disease conditions which we trace, or should trace, to absorption of bacteria. In the absence of pyorrhea, other inflammatory conditions of equal importance may exist in the mouth.

There are many varieties of infectious condition of the mucous membrane, which will be dealt with in the following chapters. Hunter [2] has stated that Tonsillitis is very frequently the result of mouth infection; and the probable cause is infected sockets, membranes and abscessed teeth, the drain of which continually passes over these glands.

A mouth which abounds in tooth decay, stomatitis, gingivitis and pyorrhea alveolaris is a perfect menstruum for the development of bacteria. It is reasonable to charge to this condition, otherwise diagnosed diseases, especially in so closely related organs as the tonsils. The importance of this is manifold, since many other diseases frequently result from infection of the tonsils and from pharyngitis; and other affections may follow where stomatitis or gingivitis exist.

Allan, in "Vaccine Therapy and Opsonic Treatment," says in regard to the administration of vaccines by the mouth, that favorable results were obtained in staphylococcal, streptococcal, pneumococcal and tubercular infections. This point thus arises. If vaccine can be successfully administered through the mouth, what must be expected where pus, laden with bacteria, is continually swallowed?

Latham (quoted by Allen) advocates the administration of vaccines by the mouth, on an empty stomach. He considers the absorption to be almost perfect at certain times. We must expect some absorption if bacteria and their products are continually swallowed when there is little or no hydrochloric acid in the stomach.

Hunter [3] attributes to mouth organisms; gastritis, septic fevers, profound septicaemia, anaemia, tonsillitis, and pharyngitis, to which must be added, via the tonsils, many cases of muscular and articular rheumatism. Aaron Burr [4] has laid out a plan to prevent ocular disease, by the remedy of this oral condition. Miller [5] points out various diseases, such as diphtheria, syphilis, pulmonary diseases and disorders of the digestive tract, resulting from presence of bacteria in the mouth.

The dentist is prone to discharge the patient after inserting beautiful fillings, crowns, plates and appliances for the improvement of mastication; and to overlook the pus-ridden sockets and necrosed roots; thus leaving a source of infection discharging as before. The skillful surgeon, who, in preparation for all operations on the stomach and intestinal tract, is punctilious with his scrubbing and disinfection beyond the slightest point of criticism, would consider it almost criminal to close an operation, knowing he had a drop of pus in the wound, yet many to-day, are paying no heed to the disinfection of the oral cavity prior to an operation.

Miller and others have shown that the pathological organisms can be killed in the mouth by proper sterilization, yet this is not sufficient, for this is only temporary asepsis and the treatment must be kept up a sufficient length of time.

In diagnosing gastric disorders the absence of proper teeth for mastication has been taken into consideration as an afterthought, and it was considered as detrimental in the disease. Tooth destruction was considered a result of regurgitated ferments from the stomach. This, however, is the crudest conception, these conditions should be considered as the cause and not the result of the gastric disorders.

Treatment and Sterilizating

As described in Chapter Two, calcareous deposits should be removed, teeth cleaned and polished, all spaces being cleaned by floss, rubbers, etc., roots extracted and the sockets which are flowing with pus should be sponged out with a solution of listerine, 5 per cent, phenol or Dobell's solution in hot water. The writer has had success in using tincture of iodine, placed on a pledget of cotton and forced to the bottom of these sockets, the cotton being removed at once and followed with proper syringing. Necrosed alveoli should be scraped and particles removed.

For painful sockets a pledget of cotton saturated with campho-phenique or tincture of calendula is used to good advantage; or a thin paste of orthoform and iodoform, equal parts, made with campho-phenique may be used; the pledget being left in the socket for twelve hours. When the mouth has been treated in this way, if the edges of the gums around the teeth are very much inflamed, it is well to paint these raw surfaces with a 5 or 10 per cent, solution of resorcin, a saturated solution of tannic acid in tincture of iodine, or a good counter-irritant. Then in twenty-four hours it will be well to have the patient use the brush with a little powdered pumice once or twice, as directed in the following chapter, and continue the mouth wash, allowing plenty of time for the antiseptic action of the solution.

[1] "Micro-organisms of the Human Mouth." - Miller.
[2] "Oral Sepsis," Hunter.
[3] "Oral Sepsis," Hunter.
[4] "Dental Cosmos," July, 1910.
[5] "Micro-organisms of the Human Mouth," Miller.

Chapter Two - Salivary Deposits

When the patient comes for emergency treatment, it is because he has suffered. In many cases, this is the only reason why he seeks relief or treatment. Our first duty is to give him relief. The various conditions with their emergency treatment will be taken up by subjects in the succeeding chapters. The following chart shows the percentage of men who were treated by the writer during a recent period, the ages ranging from 18 to 35 years, where salivary calculus was present in each case and who were asked the question: "Do you clean your teeth?" Having treated these men, the veracity of the small percentage who claim they clean their teeth, is doubted.

Patients treated	a	b	c	d	Total
540	99	72	21	348	540

Explanation. — Teeth cleaned
  a. Three times daily.
  b. Once a day.
  c. Once a month.
  d. Never cleaned.

This percentage of patients who come for emergency treatment is met with in every day practice.

When a patient presents himself with fetid breath, swollen, bleeding gums and large masses of deposits on the teeth, with no individual tooth aching, there is evident lack of care and the condition demands emergency treatment. There are two distinct kinds of deposits, or tartar (as it is sometimes called) on the teeth. The two most frequent locations for it are just behind and on the lower margins of the lower incisors, joining and impinging on the gums, and on the buccal or cheek side of the upper molars. This is caused by the proximity of the ducts of salivary glands, the sub-maxillary and sub-lingual for the lower incisors and the parotid glands for the molars.

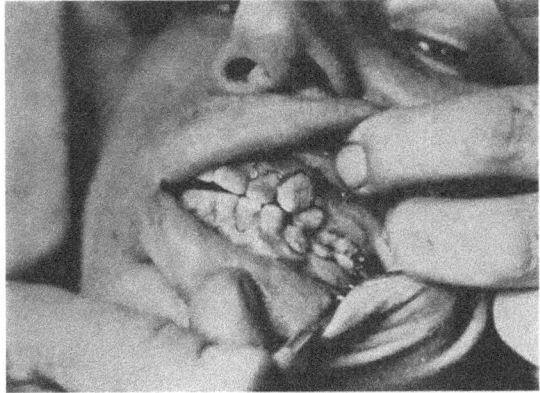

Fig. 1. — Salivary calculus on the right side of the mouth where teeth were all in place and occlusion would be normal, were calculus removed. Presented for pain on this side of the mouth. Result of neglect.

The deposition of tartar is not a normal condition, as it is seldom found in wild animals, or people like the Indians, who use their teeth with gross food, so it naturally follows that the kinds of food we use, lack of exercise of the organs, and lack of care, account largely for its presence.

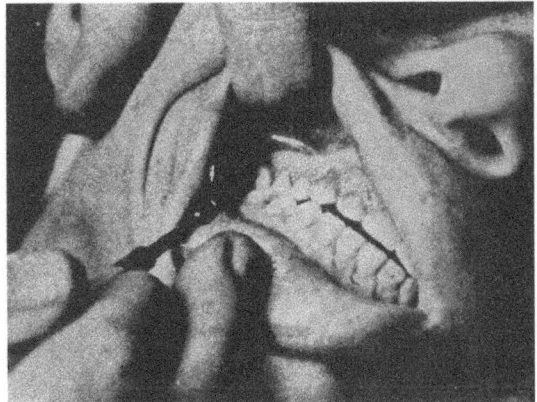

Fig. 2. — Opposite side of same mouth, one tooth missing, absence of calculus because of use for mastication.

As stated above, there are two kinds of tartar, viz., serumal and salivary. Serumal, as the name implies, is deposited from the serum of the blood and is always originally located under the free margins of the gums, where the blood supply, coming into contact with the tooth, deposits it. This is the form found in patches or small rings on the sides and necks of the teeth. Some writers believe it to be the most dangerous class, because it is very hard and irritating to the peridental membrane and is believed to play a large part in the etiology of pyorrhea alveolaris.

Salivary calculus is, as the name implies, derived from saliva, the analysis of which is as follows (quoted from Tome's "Dental Surgery"):

Salivary Calculus

Earthy phosphate	79.0
Salivary mucus	12.5
Ptyalin	1.0
Animal matter in hydrochloric acid	7.5

Salivary deposits are found in great quantities in neglected mouths. The writer has removed masses which have completely covered a tooth, no opposite tooth occluding. Not only is the deposit of tartar to be taken into consideration, but where there are large patches, under the margin and in the shelf formed by them and the gum will be found a veritable hot-bed of bacteria, and in all probability some formation of pus. If there is an inflammation and irritation of the alveolar process, this emergency demands your attention. The bacteriological aspect resulting from this condition, and the mouth in general, has been taken up in another chapter.

It is the intention of the writer to make plain the treatment, the methods and the instrumentation for removing deposits, which will relieve the immediate condition presented.

The proper removal of deposits is not a simple matter and to successfully clean away this irritating substance will test the skill of a good operator. The description of a simple method of relieving this condition, will, however, be attempted.

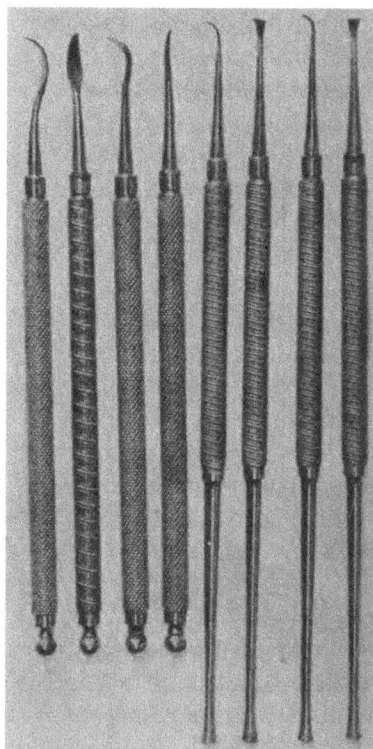

Fig. 3. — Four scalers which can be used with success in removal of deposits on the teeth (side and front view).

There are two principal plans of procedure for removal of deposits, the push cut and the draw cut methods. [1] Only the draw cut method will be suggested in this chapter. The daily use of the push cut method renders the process easy, but the occasional use of this method is not advised. The draw cut method does not alarm the patient because he feels you are drawing the instrument away from the sensitive tissues. The scalers in Fig. 3 are photographed from two views, showing the shape, form and cutting edges. These four instruments will, if diligently applied, render relief in all cases presented for emergency treatment. Grip the instrument with the thumb and first finger while the second finger forms a guard or fulcrum; then holding the instrument beneath the calculus, draw it on the long axis of the tooth away from the gums.

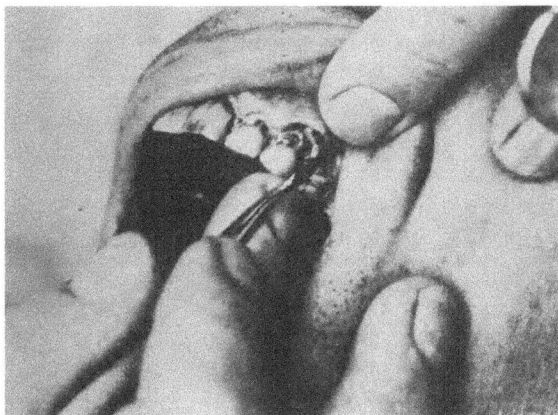

Fig. 4. — Method and position of the instrument and fingers for removing deposits from the upper incisors. The position of the second finger of right hand will be noted as forming a fulcrum.

Figs. 4 to 8 demonstrate the position and protection of the lips, etc., with the left hand during this process.

There is no fear of cavities under these deposits of salts, because their presence must have resulted from the existence of an alkaline reaction and we have no caries except in acid reaction.

Patients firmly believe at times, that cavities must exist on the lower anterior teeth where deposits have

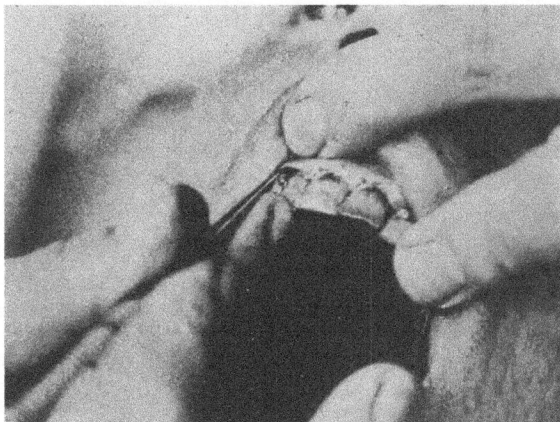

Fig. 5. — Method of removing deposit from upper right side of mouth, showing protection of lips with left hand.

pushed the gums away and exposed the peridental membrane. This at times is very sensitive and too much force on the instrument, with too much pressure against the tooth, should be avoided. There is no possibility of removing the enamel with the deposit, because it is merely a foreign matter attached to the enamel; and while it clings in many cases, it will be removed by perseverance and proper instrumentation. The engine with bristle brushes and wooden poitits, rubber cups, etc., is ordinarily used after all the deposits have been removed, but this being only an emergency, the medicinal treatment should now be applied.

11

Paint the edges of the gums, when they are inflamed with resorcin, 10 per cent, solution, tincture of iodine, or the counter-irritant tincture of iodine, tincture of aconite and chloroform equal parts; then give the patient a good antiseptic mouth wash. Instruct him how to use it in hot water, holding a quantity of same in the mouth, for a few minutes each time used, and on the following day to massage the gums with the fingers. Then on the second day, have him use a small quantity of powdered pumice stone as a tooth powder and give the instructions on care of the teeth. Cleaning, not medicine and fancy mouth washes, aids nature most in reverting to the normal conditions. Instruct the patient in properly brushing the teeth, to place the bristles of the brush on the gums and by a downward or rotary movement of the hand, bring the bristles over the teeth. For the lower, the bristles will be placed on the gums and an upward or circular movement will give the same result, completing a circle with the brush. Then brush over the cutting edges and inside by the straight in and out motion. For the inside of the lowers use a lift movement of the bristles and brush the cutting surfaces, the same as the upper. Use floss silk for removing particles of food between the teeth, where the contact points are bad and

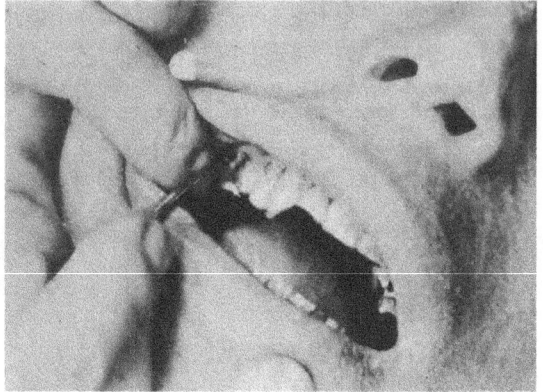

Fig. 6. — Showing position of instrument and first finger of left hand which prevents instrument from slipping and injuring the gums.

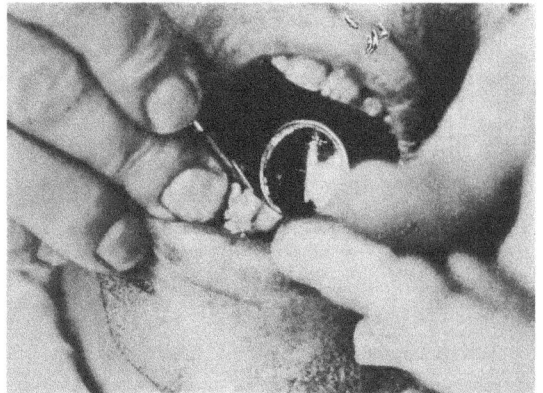

Fig. 7. — Position for removal of deposits from inner surface of lower central with use of the mirror.

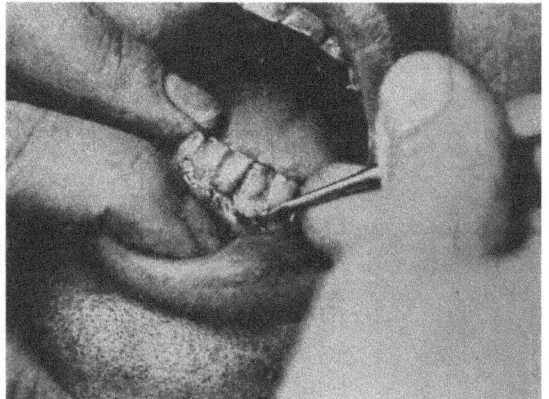

Fig. 8. — Position of the instrument in removal of deposits from labial or outer surfaces of lower centrals, showing protection of the lips and fulcrum formed by second finger.

strands of food are held. Do not snap the floss silk down and injure the gums, in the interproximal spaces. The use of the wooden toothpick is injurious and absolutely unwise, as it works great havoc with the gums and the peridental membrane of the teeth. In case any pick is used, the quill is permissible, being soft and pliable and there is no chance of splinters being left to injure the gums.

Many powders, liquids and paste tooth preparations on the market are more detrimental than nothing at all. A good paste makes the habit of cleaning the teeth more attractive and pleasant. The main point, however, in all, is the proper use of the tooth brush with plenty of water.

[1] "Principles and Practice of Filling Teeth," Johnson.

Chapter Three - Inflammation of The Mucous Membrane of the Mouth

Stomatitis. — A catarrhal inflammation of the mucous membrane of the mouth, which is divided etiologically into many classes. Marshall makes a classification as follows: u stomatitis simplex, stomatitis catarrhal, stomatitis apthosa, stomatitis parasitica and stomatitis ulcerosa." This classification meets the demands of differential diagnosis very well indeed; however, only the local conditions, as a whole, will be dealt with in this chapter.

The various causes of stomatitis are both local and constitutional. Among the local irritants are bad-fitting plates, bridges, crowns and fillings, and rough edges causing irritation; also unhygienic conditions in bottle-fed children. Constitutional causes include malnutrition, conditions caused by unhealthy quarters, various diseases which alter the condition of the blood, as scarlet fever, diphtheria, scrofula; effects of medicines, such as the use of mercury, etc. There can be no doubt that parasitical conditions of the mouth enter into this etiology.

The surgeon in charge of the case should be consulted, as to the systemic condition. Its treatment, from this standpoint, should always be directed by him, especially as to changes of treatment causing this condition.

Ill-fitting plates, bridges, crowns or fillings should be removed and not replaced in the mouth until the conditions are healed or repaired.

The local treatment of nearly all cases should be as follows: The mouth should be irrigated with boric acid solution, Dobell's solution or other mild antiseptic, with a wash at some stage, always, of potassium chlorate, gr. v, to the ounce of water. Surfaces with glistening patches coalescing until the whole mucous membrane seems covered should be treated with emmolient lotions, such as borax and honey, glycerine, weak solution of acetate of lead, gr. iii, to the ounce of water, or a very weak solution of alum. A few doses of potassium bromide will relieve the nervous condition. [1]

A great many men who live in barracks and eat the same prepared food will, at times, seem to present an epidemic, which is simple stomatitis. The irritated parts should be touched with resorcin, 10 per cent, or tincture of iodine. If the patient be given a good cathartic and advised to refrain from the eating of meats, and given a glass of good strong lemonade, twice daily, for about three days, the normal condition will generally return.

Herpes Labialis (Fever Blisters) . — An acute inflammatory affection, characterized by the formation of vesicles, or groups of same, on the skin or mucous membrane.

Herpes is called fever blisters, also "cold sores," these names arise from the etiology, being frequent in all kinds of fevers and when the patient is suffering from a cold or intestinal indigestion.

Forming blisters on the lips, they are very liable to be broken, and when they are they become very painful. The adjustment of the rubber dam and all other dental work over the lips, which might injure or bruise the tissues, cause their appearance and they may persist and recur, because some patients are of a herpetic diathesis.

Treatment

Clean the affected part with alcohol or hydrogen peroxide and apply oil of cloves, or campho-phenique (the latter being much preferred).

A large sore which is liable to break and bleed may be kept soft by the use of zinc oxide ointment. Very painful sores result from the vesicles breaking and from exposure to the wind, etc., and these raw surfaces should be washed clean with hydrogen peroxide or alcohol and then seared with campho-phenique and a thin layer of cotton placed over the part and this covered with Collodium.

Canker "Sore Mouth." — Canker sores are very small, angry ulcers with a coating of whitish yellow over the surface. The size varies from that of a grain of wheat to a pea. They are generally located on the tongue, at its junction with the ground or floor of the mouth, as well as on the buccal surfaces at the duplicature of gums and buccal membrane. They vary in depth according to the stage of progress and are always painful, they are generally round and the margins well defined, but these must not be confused with the more perfectly defined margins of the chancrous ulcer. The membrane around the ulcer is always red and inflamed. Pressure within an inch will cause pain at the point of contact. The writer has observed them to appear suddenly in men, especially after excessive or unaccustomed use of alcoholic beverages, and they are common in pregnant women, appearing and reappearing.

Authors differ as to the cause of canker sore mouth, many believe their origin to be solely in the mouth while others attribute their cause to trophic disturbances. [2] The duration, characteristic appearance, size, pain, and location of these ulcers renders diagnosis comparatively easy.

Treatment

The mouth should be washed out with a good antiseptic mouth wash (the writer prefers it made with hot water, always), such as listerine, Dobell's solution, or 5 per cent, carbolic acid solution with a few drops of the oil of gualtheria or cassia, dissolved in alcohol, added; this held in the mouth for a minute or two. The ulcer should then be washed with a pledget of cotton saturated with peroxide and the whitish-gray surfaces cleared off; the part should then be dried with alcohol and touched with a 10 per cent, solution of nitrate of silver, which cauterizes .deeply enough, but does not penetrate too far, because of the forming of a firm coagulation. [3] A pledget of cotton saturated with pure carbolic acid will also be found very useful. The writer, after using one of these applications generally paints the inflamed area immediately around the ulcer with tincture of iodine, or iodine, aconite and chloroform, equal parts. The patient will be relieved immediately by this method and seldom requires a second treatment. The mouth wash should be continued for from twenty-four to forty-eight hours.

Injuries of the Mucous Membrane

Very severe injuries to the mucous membrane; inflamed, swollen patches and surfaces present; which are the result of injuries to the tissues. The bristles of the tooth brush, may penetrate under the margins of the gums, or any other part with which the brush comes into contact in cleaning, and result in this condition to the extent of forming an abscess. This may be mistaken for an abscess of the tooth, or a "pyorrhea alveolaris socket." The writer recently treated a patient, a young lady, who had been under treatment for six months for supposed dentoalveolar abscess of the upper right central incisor. It was considered incurable and she was advised to have the tooth removed. Careful exploration showed the pus coming from the side of the root, and presence of some foreign substance under the gums about the middle of the root, which could not be removed. Incision was made opposite this point and a pus pocket opened. The contents were examined and a coarse bristle from the toothbrush found. The abscess was treated, drained and closed, and the root filled, with resultant complete disappearance of condition.

A hair, a bristle, a piece of a wooden toothpick, or a seed or any foreign substance of this class, may be found to be the cause of this painful condition.

Treatment

Removal of the foreign substance and the part washed with a warm mouth wash and touched with tincture of iodine, or aconite, iodine and chloroform, equal parts, on a pledget of cotton, will effect a cure.

Smokers' Sore Mouth. — Many excessive smokers will present large, swollen, very red, dry patches on the roof of the mouth, extending over the palate, which are extremely painful, in reality blisters.

Treatment

Wash the mouth with a warm solution of carbonate or bicarbonate of soda, or magnesia water, dry the surfaces affected with a pledget of cotton saturated in alcohol, then paint the surface with glycerite of tannin. Let the patient hold a 5-grain tablet of chlorate of potassium in his mouth until it dissolves, not chewing it, then in two hours, another one, and after that he will be able to smoke. If not repeat the treatment.

Gingivitis. — Gingivitis is an inflammation of the gums and when the margins are so affected as shown in Fig. 9, it is designated as "marginal gingivitis."

In nearly all cases where marginal gingivitis, exists, we have a subsequent degeneration of the pericementum, the membrane of attachment of the roots of the teeth to the socket. This condition is almost certain, unless proper treatment is instituted, to result in a gingivitis of the deeper tissues and interstitial gingivitis, [4] as Talbot has wisely called the condition commonly known as pyorrhea alveolaris.

Marginal gingivitis may be caused by local irritation, local infection and general effects of various origin, unhygienic quarters, food, general debility, disease, drugs, such as mercury, etc.; gonococcus bacteria are claimed to have been found in some forms of gingivitis.

In the case shown in Fig. 9, the patient had recently recovered from typhoid fever and showed absolute neglect of his teeth and mouth. Plaques of deposit, crowned the necks of all the teeth, these were covered by soft masses of decayed food, lying unmolested in a fermenting condition, far from the disturbances of mastication. The resistance to the treatment of this condition was proof of systemic involvement and bacteriological infection, aided by local irritation of deposits and food wedged between the teeth.

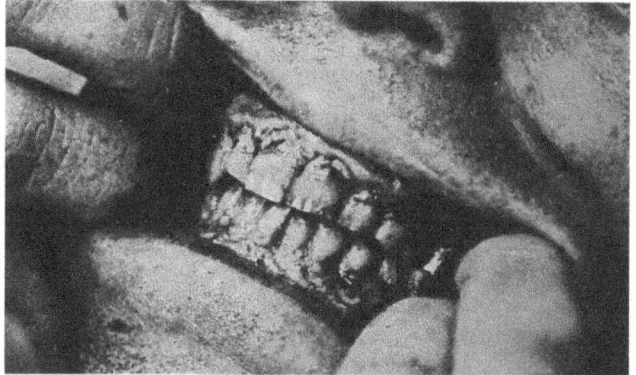

Fig. 9 — Marginal gingivitis; the result of neglect of teeth. Patient recently dismissed from hospital, case of typhoid fever. Mouth had not been treated or cared for, by his statement and by appearance.

Marginal gingivitis appears at the necks of the teeth, presenting a red, swollen, inflamed surface, which bleeds with the slightest touch, the gums are easily raised away from the deposit and are raw and very painful.

Salivary deposits are generally present or some other mechanical object of irritation, such as ill-fitting crowns, fillings, plates, bridges, etc., or the existence of bad contact points, which permit the food to lie unmolested between the teeth and result in a fermentation, irritating the gums to inflammation. Too violent brushing of the teeth and the use of too strong astringent mouth washes, will also cause the inflammation.

When gingivitis appears in more than one or two places, that is, a general gingivitis on the margins of all of the teeth, it is usually the result of local irritation, salivary deposits.

These irritated points form shelves between the margins of the gums and the tartar and present an ideal location for the fermentation of food, as well as an injured raw surface, open to the attack of the oral bacteria. The gums, pushed away from the necks of the teeth, are very spongy, very much swollen and congested, with irregular attachments to the teeth; and at times present a purple appearance, indicating excessive congestion.

This condition treated and proper care of the mouth given by the patient will prevent subsequent development of the more serious and positive interstitial gingivitis or pyorrhea alveolaris.

Treatment

Local treatment will ease the condition and prevent further developments, unless an underlying constitutional condition is the cause. The following treatment will aid and be necessary even in the presence of the correction of this condition. Wash the mouth with a warm solution of half and half Dobell's solution and water; 5 per cent, phenol, or a weak solution of potassium permanganate or a solution of the mouth wash given below, then with the same method as employed in the removal of deposits, as shown in Figs. 4 to 8, remove the calculus and food debris from around the necks of the teeth and again flush out the sockets which appear at the margins. The gums will be very tender and tear, almost at the touch of the instrument; but care will prevent this to any great extent and the profuse bleeding will help reduce the congestion. Take an orange wood stick, preferably, trim it to a flat surface and paint the rough raw surfaces with a 10 per cent, solution of trichloracetic acid, this will tend to reduce and astringe these affected surfaces. With a pledget of cotton, saturated with tincture of iodine, paint over all the affected parts.

Give the patient a good mouth wash, such as:

R. Boroglycerinae, [5]
Tinct. of krameriae,
Tinct. of calendulae,
Alcoholis...āā 30 c.c.

17

Sig. — Two tablespoonfuls to a glass of water several times daily.

The writer has found this wash to have a very curative effect upon the injured tissues. Let the patient use this for one day after treatment, then proper care and brushing of the teeth, will, in most cases, prevent a recurrence.

[1] "Dental Medicine," Gorgas.　　　[4] "Interstitial Gingivitis," Talbot.
[2] Pusey: quoted by Buckley.　　　[5] Burchard and Inglis.
[3] Prinz.

Chapter Four - Syphilis in the Mouth

Syphilis will be dealt with, not from the standpoint of the general practitioner, treating the case, constitutionally, but from that of the dental operator. Too much emphasis cannot be placed upon its importance to those who operate with the object of dental relief.

Some men in the past have felt that they should not treat dental cases, where syphilitic symptoms were present or suspected. In our province of relieving pain, we cannot admit to a patient that we are not sufficiently cautious, skillful and informed to successfully treat him without infecting ourselves or our other patients.

First-aid treatment in these cases, is as necessary and at times, more gratifying, than in many others. The writer's experience has been that syphilitics are exceedingly pleased to have rubber gloves used and all other precautions taken in treating their cases. One of the most agonizing cases of dental suffering the writer has ever treated, was a syphilitic, presenting abscessed teeth and necrosed roots, immediately under a large oozing mucous patch. The practice advocated by some men, of the destruction of instruments after using in suspected syphilis, is expensive, useless, and foolish; since a good scrubbing with green soap and boiling in a sterilizer for not less than fifteen minutes, will suffice to make sure of asepsis.

When we know that the patient has syphilis and he comes for dental treatment, precautions must be taken, yet the value of extra precaution must be considered in all patients, because we do *not* ordinarily know that patients are syphilitic. Syphilis is not a respecter of persons, sex, age, position or society and patients the least suspected may carry the spirochaeta of the scourge.

Primary Syphilis

The primary lesion of acquired syphilis appears from ten to ninety days, an average of twenty-one days after, and at the point of, infection. Appearing as an eroded, hard papule, losing its coating after a few days, it is raw, ulcerated and surrounded by a tough, hard ring. The lesion is called the chancre *and is painless.* The lymphatic glands lying in adjacent parts become swollen.

The important point in this work is the extra-genital chancre, which appears so frequently on the lips, in the mouth, on the fingers, etc., and may be the direct result of ignorance or neglect in the care of instruments, appliances and the hands of the operator. Keyes gives a table of seventy cases of extra-genital chancres, which will serve to emphasize the importance of this fact by the various locations given:

Cases

Males 70	Cheek 1	Tongue 4	Arm 1
Tonsils 2	Lip 24	Eyelid 1	
Finger 34	Chin 1	Abdomen 2	

Keyes states that almost all the finger infections are of doctors, due to contact with affected parts. Care of the hands as well as protection of patients is again emphasized. The treatment is constitutional and within the province of the general practitioner.

Secondary Syphilis

The secondary manifestations of syphilis will generally be observed in and about the mouth, irrespective of the location of the initial chancre. These are not local infections, but the result of the general progress of the disease. The eruptions of this stage are found alike on the skin and the mucous membrane. Certain organs may show the result of acute inflammation. At the time of the fevers accompanying the eruptions, mucous patches occur on the mucosa of the mouth and in any part of the oral cavity. The pharynx and the larynx are also affected by the inflammation. The copper-colored areas (like pus seen through a membrane over the point of a boil) appear under the outer mucous lining, on some part of the membrane of the lips, palate, buccal or labial regions, pharynx or tonsils. They soon break down and form the mucous patches which are the most virulent and dangerously infectious lesions of the disease.

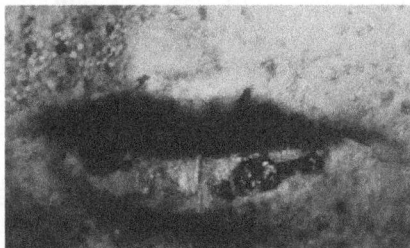

Fig. 10 — Typical case of herpes labialis. (Cold sores or fever blisters.)

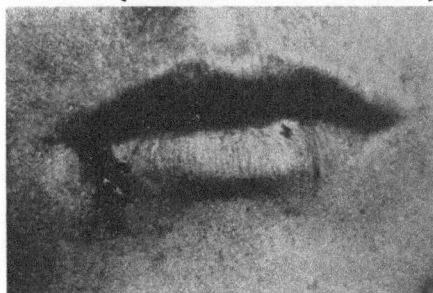

Fig. 11 — Syphilitic chancre. The one on the reader's right was full of pus just under the outer mucous membrane — the black spot indicates the yellow pus in the tissue.

19

This condition is of paramount importance to the operator on the oral cavity, as the lesion can, at times, scarcely be diagnosed from the ordinary "fever blisters" (herpes labialis). Illustrations No. 10 and No. 11 show two cases which the writer treated for dental pain on the same day. Compare the vicious, painful patch of Herpes with the more innocent appearing, painless mucous patch. Diagnosis of this condition at any time must be determined by other signs of syphilis, in other parts of the body, as enlarged glands, skin eruptions, areas of papular eruption on the membrane of the throat; also other signs, as falling out of hair, eyebrows, etc. Frequently a diagnostic sign is that of indefinitely located dental pain. [1] The point of importance for the dental operator is to be able to determine these conditions and to take precautions for his patient's and his own protection; to refer the case to a general practitioner for systemic treatment if the patient is not under his care at the time.

The use of mercury in these cases, is almost universal; even with the present use of salvarsan, mercury is and should be used as a following treatment. The appearance of ptyalism has been much reduced by the new combination. However, a prophylactic treatment of the oral cavity limits the possibility of ptyalism, and mercury can be pushed much further without salivation if the mouth has been placed in a proper condition.

Tertiary Syphilis

The lesions of secondary syphilis are confined principally to the mucous and dermal tissues but the lesions of the tertiary stage arise in the deeper connective tissues and the periosteum, most often attacking the bones with thin portions, such as the bones of the skull, palate, palatal process [2] and the alveolar process.

Tertiary lesions will be noted by the oral operator in the form of ulcers, which appear first on the soft, then on the hard palate, on the lips, and on the tongue. They make their appearance usually as nodes under the skin or mucous membrane, and become larger as they approach the surface and break gradually through, forming an ulcer. This may perforate the palate and the extensive necrosis will at times totally destroy the bones of the surrounding parts. The more frequent affection in the mouth, however, is the bone of the upper jaw. When the lower bone is affected, according to Marshall, it is generally in the alveolar process. He states a case where the palatal bones, the nasal bones and nearly the entire upper jaw, were destroyed, the soft palate being intact.

These ulcers are malignant in the extreme and attack, impartially, every organ. Under treatment, systemic or local, they have very little tendency to disappearance. Authorities differ as regards the possibilities of infection from these lesions. Keyes states that "they are clinically not infectious." However, an ugly, stubborn ulcer in the mouth of a patient should be looked upon with great caution and the same care be taken in operating and sterilizing, etc., as with other stages. Trauma, such as injury of dental tissues in treating the pulps of teeth, abscesses, pyorrhea alveolaris, extractions, etc., may be the cause of extensive necrosis in cases with a history of syphilis. It does not matter what has been the result of its treatment and the confidence of its cure.

In case of accidental infection from an instrument used on a syphilitic patient, an ointment composed of ten parts of calomel and twenty parts lanolin, applied by inunction to the infected part, will probably prevent syphilitic infection if used within one hour of the inoculation. Mercuric chloride is claimed to be of no avail. [3]

Differential Diagnosis of Chancre and Herpes (Taken from Keyes)

Syphilitic Chancre

1. History: Sexual contact, kissing, mediate infection, vaccination, etc.
2. Incubation: Two to six weeks. None.
3. Commencement. Begins as an erosion or papula and remains an erosion or ulcerates.
4. Number: Usually unique or simultaneously multiple, rarely multiple by successive crops by successive auto-inoculation, never confluent.
5. Physiognomy:
(a) Shape: round, oval or symmetrically irregular.
(b) Lesion: is habitually flat, capped by erosion or superficial ulceration; or scooped out, or a deep funnel-shaped ulcer with sloping edges. Sometimes the papula is dry and scaly.
(c) Edges: sloping and adherent. Sometimes prominently elevated.
(d) Bottom: smooth, shining.
(e) Color: somber, darkish red, gray or black, sometimes livid and scaly, occasionally scabbed.
(f) Secretion: slight, serosanguinolent, unless irritation provokes suppuration.
8. Induration: Constant, parchment like and very faint, or cartilaginous and extensive, terminating abruptly not shading off into parts around; movable upon parts beneath the skin and not adherent to the latter, outlasts the sore and remain for months usually.
9. Sensitiveness: Absent.
10. Duration: At least a fortnight.

Herpes

1. History: Relapsing herpes.
2. Incubation: None.
3. Commencement. Begins as a group of vesicles, rarely as a single vesicle, and becomes an ulcer.
4. Usually multiple simultaneously and by successive crops of vesicles sometimes confluent.

(a) Shape: irregular, rounded with borders describing segments of small circles left by confluent vesicles.

(b) Lesion: usually superficial, sometimes in solitary Herpes there is but one absolutely circular vesicle. There are usually neighboring vesicles to clear up the diagnosis.

(c) Edges: sharp, not undermined.

(d) Bottom: even, inflammatory.

(e) Color: like chancre.

(f) Secretion: slight, seropurulent.

8. Induration: inflammatory, capable of being produced by some cause as in the chancroid and behaving in a precisely similar manner.

9. Sensitiveness: Beginning, heat.

10. Duration: Rarely more than ten days.

Ptyalism (Salivation)

In the treatment of syphilis, the administration of mercury is necessary in more than the tonic dose. In many cases the patient must be poisoned to cure the lesion. Mercury is an alterative and tonic in small doses but in severe cases of syphilis it is pushed far beyond this point. Mercurialism as shown by the gums, or mild salivation, indicates the stopping of its administration. The stopping of the mercury will, in these mild cases, affect a cure. Mercury has a selective influence on the gums, jaws and adjacent parts. [4] In more severe cases, the first symptoms noticed by the patient are a coppery, metallic taste in the mouth, fetor of the breath, inflammation of the gums and swollen tongue, showing the imprint of the teeth. The gums bleed freely and a severe pericementitis of the teeth is present, with much pain when the jaws are forcibly closed. If the drug is not withdrawn, the condition grows worse, saliva flows from the mouth, there is drooling and the tongue swells, teeth become so loose in the sockets that they may be picked out with the fingers (they should not be extracted, however). The glands swell and ulcerations occur in the mouth. Mercurial ulceration appears behind the lower incisors and back of the lower wisdom teeth; finally the soft tissue sloughs and necrosis of the bone sets in and sequestra form, whose subsequent removal is necessary.

Treatment

The care of the mouth for the prevention of salivation has been described above. Any patient who is to be given a course of treatment with mercury should have all irritating crowns, bridges, or plates repaired or removed, all roots extracted and be instructed to be conscientious in the brushing of his teeth and gums properly, at least three times daily; and be given a mouth wash, such as potassium chlorate, gr. xv, dissolved in half a tumbler of water, for hardening the gums.

The patient with a profuse ilow of saliva should be given refrigerating, acidulated drinks. The ulcerations may be touched with tincture of aconite, tincture of iodine, and chloroform or with:

Tinct. of Myrrh.   }
Tinct. Iodum Comp. } ....āā 4 gms.
Aquae   }

Sig: Apply to gums once or twice daily. [5]

Atropin in medicinal doses may be used by the physician in charge to control the excessive flow of saliva. The systemic treatment should not be changed except by him.

When the evidence of necrosis is at hand and the parts can be treated, Mawhinney recommends the local application of 50 per cent, solution of phenosulphic acid, which acts as a stimulant and hastens the formation of sequestra.

[1] Hugenschmidt: quoted by Burchard.

[2] Keyes.

[3] Metchinoff: quoted by Burchard and Inglis.

[4] Buckley.

[5] Buckley.

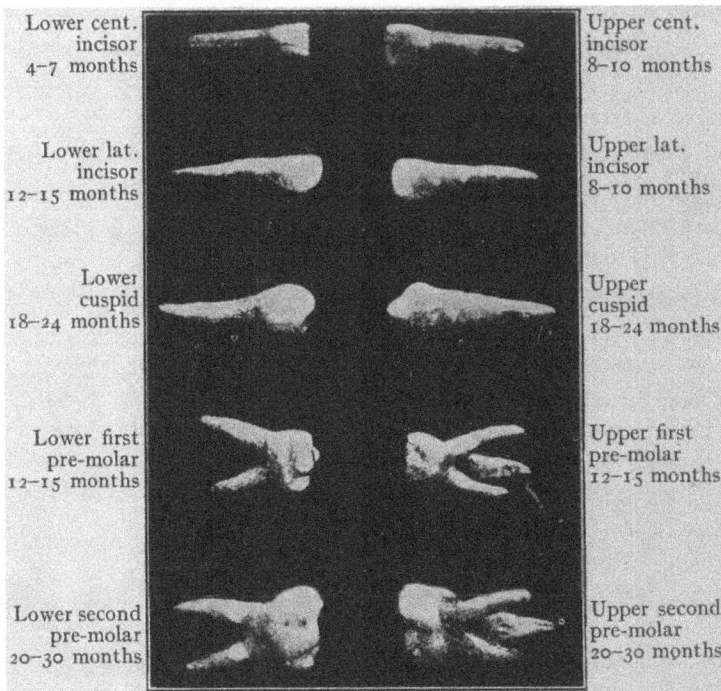

Fig. 12. — The deciduous teeth and time of their appearance (left side of mouth only). — *(From Broomell.)*

Chapter Five - Brief Dental Anatomy

In order to intelligently treat or relieve dental disturbances, it is necessary for the operator to have a knowledge of the parts, their construction, relation, organs of supply, histology and functions. It is not intended to give in this chapter a full and extensive treatise on this large and important branch, but to give a few ideas which will aid in all emergency treatments presented.

The temporary or deciduous teeth number five on each side, from the median line backward, the full set being ten in each jaw. These teeth erupt from the fifth to the thirtieth month and complete their full service with the eruption of the permanent set.

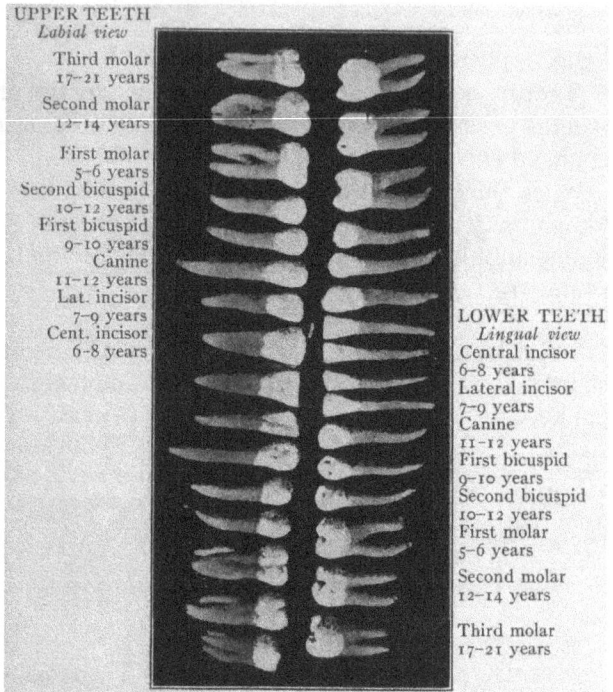

Fig. 13. — Eruption of the permanent teeth. — (From Broomell.)

The chart, Fig. 12, shows the time of eruption of the temporary teeth, and chart, Fig. 13, the eruption of the permanent teeth. Comparison of these figures and tables will show that the time of the loss of the temporary teeth is about that of the eruption of the corresponding permanent teeth.

The importance of this comparison of the relative time of loss and eruption should be seriously considered in the decision as to the advisability of extracting deciduous teeth. Premature or delayed extraction may result in a malocclusion and compel the patient, in a few years, to undergo the

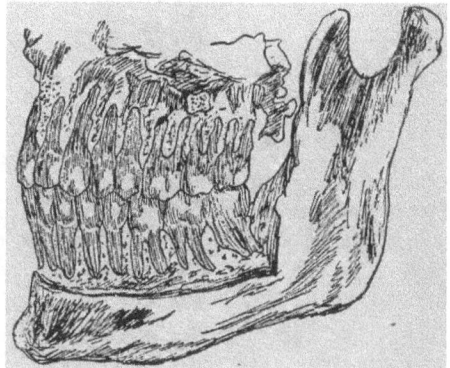

Fig. 14. — The teeth in position with extreme alveolar plate removed, showing relative position of the roots. — (Johnson.)

tedious process of regulation of the permanent set. Deciduous teeth should not be extracted when they ache any more than permanent teeth, but the treatment of the condition should be made to preserve the teeth for their full period of usefulness.

Fig. 14, by Johnson, is an excellent exhibit of the two sets of teeth *in situ.* The external plates of the alveolar process being removed, the reader is able to secure an accurate idea of the angles, position and relation of the roots of the various classes of teeth, as they normally exist.

Fig. 15 presents the diagram of the structure and implantation of the normal incisor tooth, a study

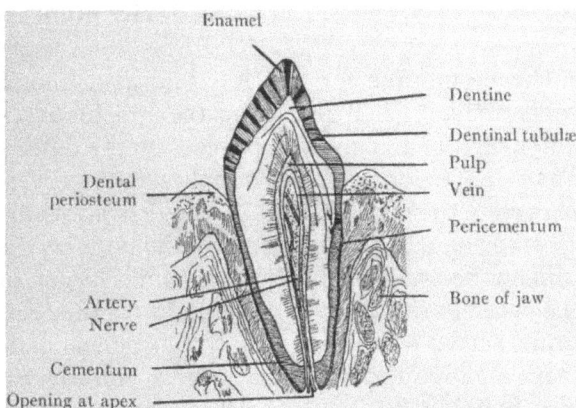

Fig. 15. — Vertical section of an incisor tooth.

of which will fix in the mind the exact anatomy and relation of the teeth. Those having multiple roots have the same histology and source of supply for each root.

The Enamel

The *enamel* is the hardest and most compact part of the tooth, the part which forms the outer exposed surface and covers the crown. It is formed in prisms or rods, lying generally parallel to each other and resting at one extremity on the dentine. The rods are held together by a very minute layer of cement substance, presenting a solid mass to the naked eye.

The Dentine

The *dentine* is the tissue which forms the principal mass of the tooth. It is a modification of bony tissue, differing, however, in that the cells lie only at the periphery of the pulp, and not throughout the mass. The dentine is formed around the chamber which encases the pulp. The mass is traversed by small canals (dentinal canaliculi) which run in a course from the pulp outward, as is shown very clearly in the figure. These canals contain a substance, called the intertubular tissue and communicate sensation from the point of stimulation to the pulp. The dentine is surrounded or covered by the enamel in the crown portion of the tooth, and the cementum in the root portion.

The Cementum

The *cementum* is the covering over the root portion of the tooth. It varies in thicknesses, overlapping the edges of the enamel at the neck, and becoming thicker over the apical portion. The cementum is truly a bone substance, and contains Haversian canals in its thicker portion, about the apex. As age advances, the cementum becomes thicker, especially on the outer border.

The Pericementum

This membrane, for such it is, affords a lining for the alveolar sockets of the roots of the teeth. It also forms the attachment between the cementum on the inner surface and alveolar process on the outer surface, both of which it nourishes, being profusely supplied with nerves and blood-vessels. The fibers from the membrane form the firm attachment of the teeth in the socket; by entering into the substance of the bone on the one side, and the cementum on the other. The pericementum is larger, or thicker at the apical end of the roots. In the powerful concussion of the teeth in mastication this membrane acts as a shock absorber, so to speak. Being quite elastic, it permits the teeth to move about in their sockets. Moreover the pericementum has a sensory function. It is the medium by which all forces applied to the tooth surface are taken up and conveyed to the brain. [1]

The important point in this brief description is the part played by this membrane in dental pain, by reason of its richly supplied nerves and blood-vessels and its functions.

The Dental Pulp

The *dental pulp,* erroneously called the nerve, occupies the chamber or pulp canal, in the center of the tooth. It is not a nerve tissue, but fibrous cellular connective tissue, and is abundantly supplied with blood-vessels and nerve fibers. These gain their entrance through the opening at the apical end of the root, or roots. As the tooth may have a different number of roots, so it must have a corresponding number of apical openings for the supply of the vessels and nerves.

The pulp serves as the menstruum for holding the odontoblasts, or dentine-forming cells, which lie at the periphery, the pulp being forced back as the process of dentine building continues, until, in old age, the pulp chambers are nearly closed and the pulp receded.

The *vessels* of the pulp are very numerous, entering the apical foramen in three or more branches 1 they form a plexus which is the cause of the profuse bleeding from the pulps, in their removal.

The nerves generally enter by one large trunk and three or four-minute branches. After pursuing a parallel course, giving off branches in the body of the pulp, they form a rich plexus beneath the edges of the developing dentine. [2] The relationship and the structure of the dental pulp must be understood, for intelligent treatment of the greatest of maladies in emergency treatment.

The Alveolar Process

The *alveolar process* of the maxillary bones, is a strong and wide ridge of bone, which forms the root sockets. The alveolar process consists of two plates, an inner and an outer; and these are connected by septa, which separate the sockets of the teeth. A process of a jaw without the teeth, looks like a solid bone, with the sockets drilled out for the respective roots of the teeth. The bone in the septa has a soft, spongy structure, very easily broken and many times septa are carried out between the roots of the teeth, in extraction. The upper edges are thin and vary in width at different teeth; viz., over the cuspid teeth, the bone is thinner than in any other part and fractures are frequently located here by reason of this fact. The process at the outer surface of the lower third molar teeth is very short and thick and at the inner surface, very thin (a point to be remembered in extractions). The reverse is practically true of the upper third molars. This process being spongy and sharp at the edges, is easily broken down, after the tooth it supports is removed.

The Gums

The *gums* are continuances of the mucous membrane of the mouth, differing from other membranes by their greater density, being composed of fibrous tissue. The gums are hard and elastic and closely connected with the periosteum of the alveolar process, seemingly a continuous tissue. The gum tissue is scantily supplied with nerves and sensibility is limited. Its ability to reconstruct or rebuild itself after injury is marked.

[1] Broomell.   [2] Tomes.

Chapter Six - Dental Pain

The pain presented being proved not to be a result of calculus, stomatitis, gingivitis, etc., of the foregoing chapters, or of pyorrhea alveolaris or neuralgia, it will be pain from the individual teeth. Toothache, in the words of the poet, Burns, "The Hell of all Diseases," to be successfully treated must be properly located and then diagnosed as to the cause when it is a simple matter to effect the cure.

There are several kinds of toothache, which are the results of various causes, which will be studied in order to accomplish what we are called upon to do.

Pulpitis
(Inflammation of the Dental Pulp)

A tooth may ache from an exposure of the pulp, where the structures have been dissolved out and undermined and the germs of decay have opened a path for various irritations to the pulp-tissue, a point of irritation and inflammation.

The pulp may also be exposed and inflamed under a leaky filling, or one which has been placed in the tooth without proper removal of decay or sterilization of the cavity.

Pulp exposures may result from the injudicious use of strong acids, which have been pumped into pockets under the gums, in the treatment of pyorrhea alveolaris. The tooth structure will be destroyed and obscure cavities form which will be very hard to find. Errors in diagnosis are very liable to occur in these cases.

Another is by mechanical abrasion, the teeth become worn and in older persons, the enamel entirely ground away, the dentine grooved and the pulp exposed. In the writer's practice, a man sixty years of age, with apparently sound teeth, from the labial view, could not close his mouth because "He felt it was close to the quick." The lingual or inner part of the upper right central was so worn and grooved by the lower that the nerve was entirely exposed.

The pulps may become exposed, also from fractures of the teeth, either by forcibly bringing the jaws together in a way to split them or by a blow. Many times a pulp will become inflamed and die without the patient knowing it, from' the result of a slight injury to a tooth.

There is another pain which we find in a live tooth, the formation of *pulp-stones,* or rather *secondary dentine, calcospherites.* The dentine cells not being forced to the periphery, mass in the body of the pulp. This is a very confusing and tedious condition to diagnose and treat. Fortunately emergency treatment except that used in pulpitis, will not be necessary.

Diagnosis
(Exposure of the Dental Pulp)

When this condition exists, the pain is such that the patient will, in most cases, have no doubt as to the tooth affected. Nevertheless, exploration should be made with a mirror and a sharp fine explorer. When the cavity is found, press the tooth gently, but firmly, with the finger and tap it with an instrument. This will not cause increased pain, because the peridental membrane is not affected. Heat, carried by means of a small piece of guttapercha, heated in an alcohol flame, held in a pair of dressing pliers, applied on the enamel, will intensify the throbbing; as will also lowering the head, since either increases the congestion of blood in the already hyperaemic pulp. A very slight amount of cold may be applied by a small stream of cold water from a syringe, where there is doubt, and this will more than intensify the pain. The history of the tooth, as to injuries, mechanical irritants and treatments of pyorrhea alveolaris, will be taken into consideration in determining this condition if the above methods fail.

Putrescent Pulp

The difference between life and death, in any tissue, organ or body, is very comprehensible and makes a great classification. In regard to the dental pulp, it is the most important point in determining the trouble and treatment. Patients will present with swollen jaws, from dento-alveolar abscess and remark that the "nerve is exposed." Such a fallacy will readily be seen, as the tooth cannot be abscessed, except by the death of the pulp. Death of the pulp is preceded by the process of inflammation. Irritation causes hyperaemia, which is one of the first causes of pain, in pulpitis. Following this, pathogenic bacteria enter and the decomposition of the pulp sets in, literally, the death.

This condition of the pulp is the beginning of various kinds of diseases. Septic pericementitis, dento-alveolar abscess, etc. By the decomposition of the complex substances of the dental pulp, two gases are formed, ammonia and hydrogen sulphid. Poisonous ptomaines and fats are also found, the result of putrefaction; this condition is the putrescent pulp.

Putrescent pulps form as a result of caries, fractures, thermal changes, teeth carrying large fillings and other conditions, which cause the irritation and inflammation of the pulp associated with infection. The gases held in the pulp-chamber, unable to escape through the tooth, result in the formation of a septic pericementitis, or a dento-alveolar abscess, by forcing septic matter through the apical opening.

Putrescence (the presence of gases) is the result of inflammatory process, with putrefaction, fermentation, and infection from bacteria, in the pulp-chamber.

Diagnosis

The anterior teeth are more easily diagnosed, when putrescent pulps exist, because there is less possibility of a partial life and death of the tissues, than in the multirooted teeth; and reflection of light through the tooth is more readily accomplished. These teeth present a bluish or brownish discoloration through the larger part of the pulp-chamber and hot instruments or gutta-percha have no effect nor has the application of cold to the surfaces of these teeth. If the cavity is open, the patient will notice a bad odor and taste from the leakage of gases and septic matter. As a rule, there is no soreness at the end of the roots, but pressure will make the patient feel, at times, the abnormal condition of the tooth, which is generally not loose. The gases which escape from these teeth, upon the opening of the chamber will be sufficient to prove the diagnosis. The odors of hydrogen sulphid and ammonia and of the putrefaction, will need only be smelled once, to be always recognized as those of a putrescent pulpchamber.

Pericementitis

Pericementitis is the inflammation of the peridental membrane of the tooth and is divided into two classes: non-septic and septic. The non-septic is caused by mechanical or drug irritants [1] such as root fillings, ill-fitting dentures, plates, crowns, bridges, the hammering in the insertion of large gold fillings,, or crowns left too long, causing a pounding on the tooth in occlusion; and drugs used in the treatment of these teeth.

Diagnosis — Non-septic Pericementitis

In *pericementitis*, not caused by the presence of septic matter or bacteria, we have an inflammation of the delicate vascular membrane which swells and enlarges and pushes the tooth slightly from the socket. The pericementum is the tactile organ of the tooth, and when inflamed it is extremely tender to percussion. The difference to be found between septic and non-septic pericementitis will generally depend upon the history of the operations on the tooth, as to the treatment and filling of the root canals. There is no pus formation in the nonseptic pericementitis. When percussion is applied, there is a dull sound; and we find a deeper color in the gum tissue. [2]

Acute Septic Pericementitis or Acute Dento-Alveolar Abscess

The septic diseases of the pericementum are almost invariably the result of infection from suppuration and gangrene of the pulp or that from the oral cavity, through the pulp chambers and root canals of dead teeth. The latter cause is most frequently a result of carelessness of the operator in forcing septic matter into the apical space with a broach. It is very questionable whether pyorrhea alveolaris pockets cause this condition, by their proximity. The writer prefers to believe this supposed condition to be an extension of the pyorrhea alveolaris itself. Acute abscesses are prone to occur under the above conditions when a patient "takes cold."

The inflammatory process is the same in the dentoalveolar region as in any other tissues of the body, the infecting organisms produce the same condition at the apex and in the apical tissues. Hyperemia follows the primary infection and sensation in the tissue is altered by the resultant pressure.

Upon the entrance of this matter into the apical tissues, and the further process of inflammation, the pain is very great because of the abnormal pressure on the sensory nerves; and the swelling of the part forces the tooth from the socket. This increases the pain and irritation, by contact with the opposite teeth. The next stage is the formation of pus by the degeneration of the apical tissues. Throbbing pains, which are extremely depressing result from the pressure of the pus-irritation and the inflammation.

The next process is the exit of the pus through the tissue which offers the least resistance; usually through the outer alveolar process, the thinnest part.

The pain is very severe during the time of this boring of the pus for an exit; but when it has accomplished the destruction at the point of advance, the pain reduces, the soft tissues offering much less resistance than the bone. There is a great difference in patients, in many the tissue will not give way so readily. Extremely large and unsightly swelling results. With abscesses on the upper teeth, the eye on the side affected becomes almost closed and the cuticle is shiny and tight.

In some cases the pus burrows through the bone and out through the gums and breaks within the mouth, without any swelling of the face. Some pus tracts will not make the exit in the mouth but will wend their way down the neck or out on the face. In many cases, the point of the abscess will not break through the mucous membrane in the mouth, which appears to be tough and resistant.

From an opening being made by lancing these abscesses will, in the majority of cases, freely discharge and evacuate the full tract. The pressure of the blood system will be evidenced by the spurts of pus with each heart beat. The formation of abscesses in patients suffering from systemic diseases may be the beginning of complications, causing the formation of necrosis of the bones, etc.

Diagnosis

In the beginning of an acute alveolar abscess the patient will feel an uncomfortable condition at the apex of the tooth, or rather in the deeper gum tissue around the tooth. He may experience reflex pains and not know which tooth is aching, but in the majority of cases presented there will be no question, the pain being localized in the tooth or directly at its apex. There is usually a smoky dark discoloration noticed, and the pressure of pus and a darkened color of the gum tissue over the roots of the tooth. No response to thermal changes will be noticed. The tooth will usually be elongated and loose, contact with other teeth being very painful and sometimes impossible. Percussion or tapping a tooth in this condition is only useful where it is not protruded or loose, as the diagnosis of the acute abscess will be fully determined by the above observations.

Chronic Alveolar Abscess

A *chronic alveolar abscess is*, as the name implies, a chronic abscess condition, in which the pus continually forms by the alternate formation and breaking down of apical tissues and granulations with the expulsion and drain of

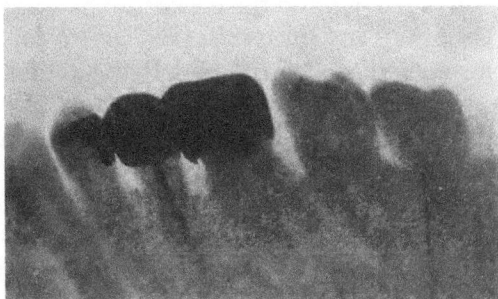

Fig. 16. — Chronic dento-alveolar abscess one root of upper, left, first molar. Radiograph. — (*Author's practice.*)

pus. The principal cause of this condition is originally the acute alveolar abscess, described above, and the causes of the former will be considered the same as those of the latter.

There are two kinds of chronic abscesses: those without an opening, except as a drain may form through the root canals of the tooth; and those which are discharging through a sinus or fistula.

The first class may drain into the mouth for months and not give the patient any pain or annoyance, because the canal of the tooth offers an exit. The drain is natural and has no resistance to its discharge; but when the root canals or pulp-chambers become stopped up and cut off the tract, swelling and reaction becomes prominent.

The chronic abscess is generally found to be on only one root of a multi-rooted tooth, all three roots of a molar, for instance, will not be affected. (See Fig. No. 16, radiograph, upper first molar.)

The tract of an abscess of this kind is lined by cicatricial tissue, which is formed in the abscess cavity and lines the tract to the end of sinus, generally on the buccal or on the outer jaw surfaces.

The tract may be compared to a blood-vessel, as the pus will lead directly from the central sac through it to the opening, the mouth of which may not be directly opposite the tooth affected. It may course down the sides of the bone and open opposite an innocent tooth. The general rule, however, is to open over the diseased tooth.

The pus in abscesses of the upper molars and bicuspids may, however, bore into the Antrum of Highmore, at the points where the bony process of its floor is thinner and offers the least resistance to the exit of the infection.

In the lower teeth, gravitation is always to be considered. The pus may bore through the body of the bone and cut on the face or chin. An impacted tooth may be the cause of a chronic abscess. With the lower wisdom teeth this is a common cause, the fistula here nearly always making its appearance through the inner plate into the mouth, or at the side of the tooth through the socket.

So much pus and the process of building up and tearing down of the new tissue, in many cases causes a necrosis of the bone, or alveolar process, at this point. It may form without the patient's being conscious of any trouble, except the appearance of a "gum boil" as he calls the teat of the fistula which recurrently fills and breaks. The complications of the chronic alveolar abscess demand attention and permanent treatment more than any other tooth affection.

Diagnosis

The stopping of the discharge of pus through the teeth, will be very difficult. When it is evaluated in treatment, it will probably persist and appear to come from an unlimited supply, which thus aids the diagnosis of the chronic condition to a great extent. The probe will pass an amazing distance through the external opening into soft tissue, without any apparent resistance, which shows the presence of destruction of the apical structure.

The diagnosis of the chronic dento-alveolar abscess is comparatively easy. When the patient has had pain in the tooth and the tract points into near-by tissue, it appears and discharges by one, two or three small openings, very close together. The use of a fine silver probe to find the direction of the tract and tooth affected will serve where there is question.

The X-ray will serve admirably here and the history of the tooth as to treatment, the pulp removed, root fillings, etc., will aid materially. The fact that it carries a filling or crown, etc., or has been treated, roots filled, only adds to the suspicion that it is the tooth affected.

[1] Buckley.   [2] Burchard.

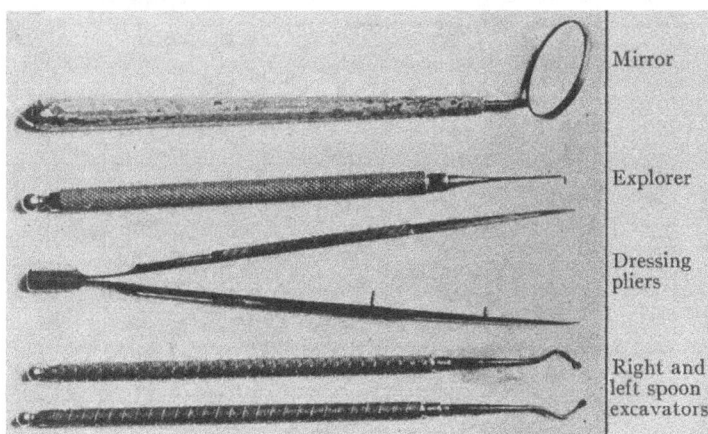

Fig. 17.

Chapter Seven - The Treatment of Pulpitis (Inflammation of the Pulp)

The first consideration in the treatment of the patient is the instruments, their care and use. Figs. 17 and 18 show the instruments which the writer believes to be necessary in the treatment of emergency cases. A mirror, dressing pliers, explorer, chisels, excavators, broaches and plastic instruments.

There should be no question in the sterilization of these instruments, they should be boiled in water a sufficient length of time and brushed clean, with the exception of the mirror. Have a clean glass or receptacle for a 10 per cent solution of formaldehyde, with a small amount of borax to prevent rust, in which to dip these instruments and to sterilize the mirror, wiping dry with a clean towel before placing in the mouth. The use of these instruments will be explained and illustrated in the following treatments. When a patient has had a severe toothache, in all probability he has neglected his teeth. Foul odors from fermenting food and a bad taste will be present and this is where we must make the sitting agreeable. A warm, body temperature solution of one of the following antiseptic mouth washes, used in a syringe, will be found to deodorize and stimulate the patient's mouth. He will feel grateful and it will be more pleasant to work in the region.

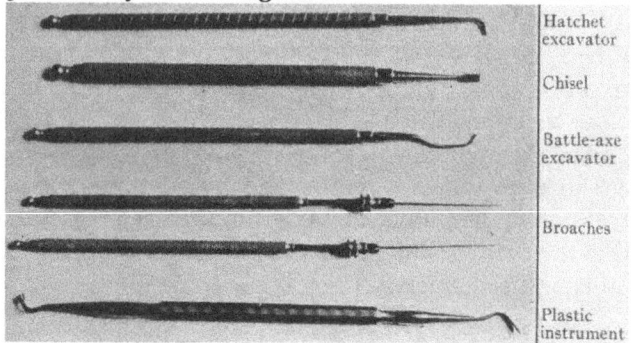

Hatchet excavator

Chisel

Battle-axe excavator

Broaches

Plastic instrument

Fig. 18.

Dobell's solution, 50 per cent, in hot water, or 5 per cent, carbolic acid, with a few drops of oil of wintergreen or cassia, dissolved in alcohol, added will make a very pleasant wash. Listerine is fairly good used in this manner. A good astringent and antiseptic is as follows:

R. Boroglycerinae,
    Tinct. krameriae,
    Tinct. Calenduale...01
    Alcoholis...āā 30 c.c.
Sig. — One or two teaspoonfuls in glass of water.

It has been said that the way to stop a tooth with an exposed pulp from aching, is to take it in out of the wet. This is correct and must be borne in mind in sealing the medicine in the cavity.

In choosing the proper drug then, we must find one that does not dissolve easily in water. For this reason cocaine or eucaine and other drugs requiring a solution to carry them or agents that are freely soluble in water, cannot be expected to keep the tooth from aching, because they wash out, although they will relieve temporarily. What we want is a drug that has anaesthetic and disinfectant properties and is

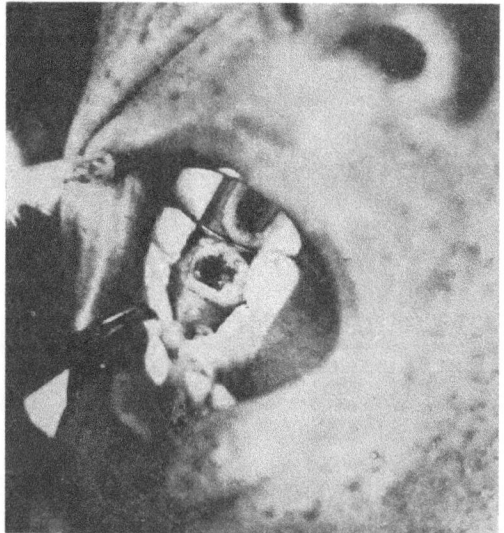

Fig. 19. — Method of excluding saliva while placing dressing in a cavity. Rolls placed on either side of tooth and held in place by mirror while the cavity is dried.

sparingly soluble in water.

The following may be used, preference in the order named: campho-phenique, carbolic acid, eugenol and oil of cloves. There are many others but this number will suffice, since the emergency case will contain at least one of the above.

The pain from which the patient is suffering having been diagnosed as pulpitis from exposure of the pulp; the preparation for its treatment will be made. The operator must be cleanly and have his hands free from dirt or infection, beyond doubt in the patient's or his own mind. Open the mouth gently, use a warm solution of a pleasant mouth wash forced through a syringe and have the parts as clean as possible. Place the mirror over the tooth and locate the cavity, then with a small pledget of cotton wipe the tooth dry as possible, observe the food particles which may be present and with a warm spray flush them from the cavity. Take two cotton rolls about the size of the second finger; place one on the outer side, between the lips or check and the gums, the other clown well between the tongue and the gum margins and hold in place by the mirror, as shown in Fig. 19. For the upper teeth, only one roll will be necessary, placed on the outside of the teeth, it will be held in place by the cheek or buccal muscles.

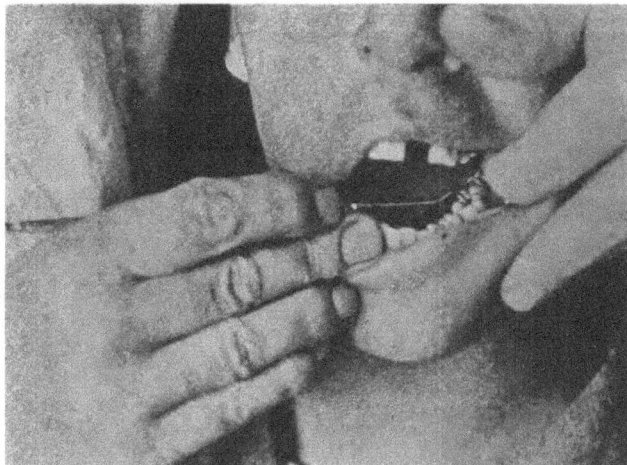

Fig. 20. — Removal of decay with spoon excavator.

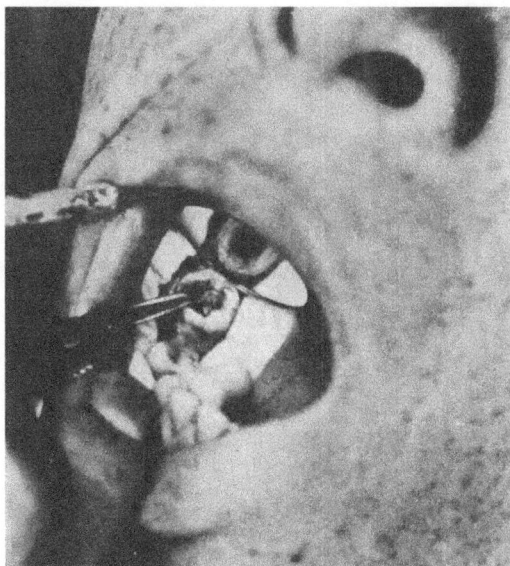

Fig. 21. — Placing medicine on pellet of cotton in the cavity of the tooth, protecting lips by ringer of hand holding tweezers.

Dry the cavity gently with cotton, and with an explorer ascertain the point of exposure. Do not force the explorer into the pulp. With a spoon excavator, shown in Fig. 20, remove the leathery decay as much as possible, drawing the instrument away from the pulp-chamber.

Dry the tooth again with a loose pledget of cotton. Prepare all the following pledgets of cotton rolled to the proper size and have the bottles containing the drugs to be used, open on a table where they are within easy reach. Saturate the first and smallest pledget in one of the above-mentioned remedies and place in the cavity as shown in Fig. 21. Then without removing the mirror, cover this with a slightly larger, loose pledget, then dip the larger one, which is slightly smaller than the cavity, in sandarac varnish or vaseline and place over the cavity. Take the first finger of the right hand and after dipping it into warm water, gently

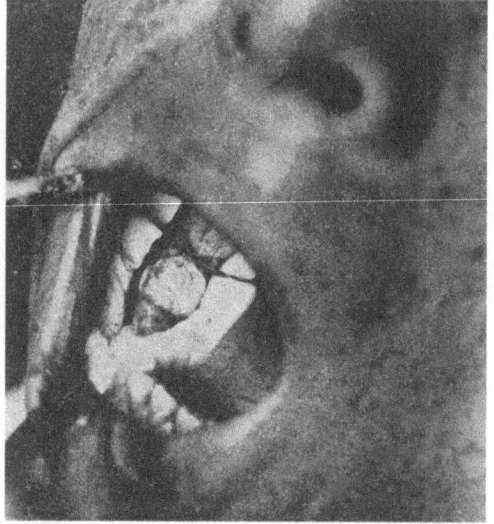

Fig. 22. — The tooth treated and medicated cotton covered by Sandaraccotton.

press the varnished or vaselined cotton as is shown in Fig. 22. Where the pulp is nearly exposed, this will be found more desirable than the use of the gutta-percha stopping, because of the difficulty in avoiding pressure, which will cause as much or more pain than before treating. Creasote should not be used in these teeth because it is supposed to be lacking in the properties desired.

In case the tooth has been aching for two days or more you will expect to find a pulp congested with blood. In

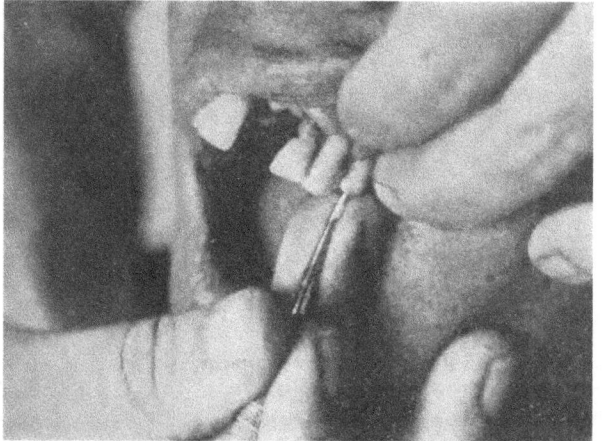

Fig. 23. — Method and position in breaking down enamel with a chisel, showing fulcrum and guard of second finger.

this case puncture the outer membrane slightly and permit the blood to ooze out. The cotton rolls and mirror being placed as described above, the bleeding can be permitted and the blood absorbed with cotton pledgets and then one of the above treatments applied.

Should the cavity be located between the teeth and the enamel be standing, but undermined, it will be necessary to take a broad chisel, as shown in Fig.

23 and break down this covering, so good access can be had to the cavity. Care must be taken to prevent the slipping of the instrument into the cavity by the guard of the second finger on the surface of the tooth as is shown in Fig. 20.

In case the exposure is not complete, the tooth should be treated in the above manner and the surface of the cavity seared with one of the drugs given, as the effect of the drug will be carried through the dentinal tubules to the pulp tissues. See Fig. 15 (Brief Dental Anatomy).

In cases where there is a filling, either firm or partially loose, difficulty will be experienced in removing it without a dental engine drill, but this can be done with chisels, in the same manner as described above in breaking down the enamel. The margins being broken, the filling is pried and lifted out with the spoon excavators, and the treatment applied as above.

When pain presents from mechanical abrasion, the enamel is worn away and the dentine is exposed or the ends of the dentinal tubules are exposed and the intertubular substance transmits irritation to the pulp.

Place cotton rolls to protect the gums and with a pledget of cotton saturated in a solution made by dissolving a small crystal of silver nitrate in a drop or two of water, sear the part. Keep the mouth open a few minutes, then remove any surplus with a cotton pledget.

Chapter Eight - The Treatment of Putrescent Pulps and Non-Septic Pericementitis

The aim of the dental operator in treating putrescent pulps is to afford an escape for gases and use a drug which will destroy or change them into a solid or liquid and prevent pressure. Buckley gives three important factors which must be accomplished, viz.: 1. Establish asepsis. 2. Prevent recurring sepsis. 3. Preserve and restore the color of the teeth. The course to be pursued by the operator in treating emergency cases, will conform to the above, except in the last point, the third factor "restore color" which will be left to the dental surgeon, not being con-

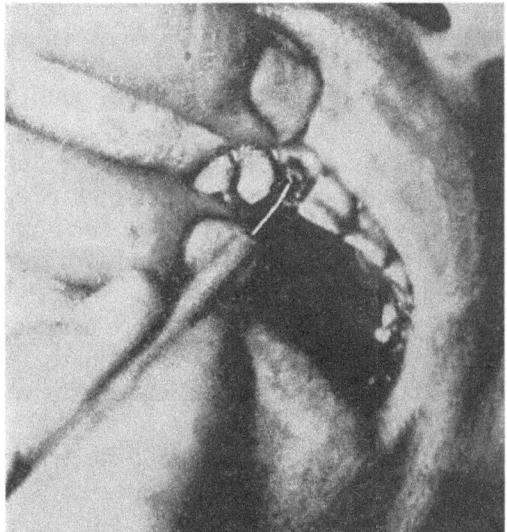

Fig. 24. — Putrescent pulp, showing manner of opening root canal mouth with a broach.

sidered an emergency.

The mouth should be treated in the same manner as described above in preparation, by flushing it out and cleaning the teeth. It is proper to apply the rubber dam over the tooth and adjoining teeth and disinfect with formalin solution, described in the preceding chapter for use in dipping instruments, but this will not usually be attempted by the operator in emergency cases.

The cotton rolls will be used as previously shown and described and the tooth will be washed with a large pledget of cotton saturated with alcohol. The opening into the pulp-chamber will now be made and the chisels described in the foregoing chapter will be used, in case the cavity has been filled and access cannot be made by the use of the excavators.

In cases where the tooth is sound and has no weak margins it will be almost impossible to make an opening without a dental engine burr, but these cases are infrequent.

The cavity being opened, the pulp-chamber should now be entered and this can easily be done, where we have access, with a spoon excavator. The opening should be large.

The chamber should be enlarged sufficiently for the mouth of the canals, as the tooth may be single or multi-rooted, to be opened by the point of the broach. Fig. 24. Do not run the instrument through the canal, merely place it in the opening to be sure that the mouth is not closed.

Take a small pledget of cotton and saturate it in the following remedy: Cresol and formaldehyde, of each equal parts. Touch it to a towel to remove the excess of the liquid and place in the pulp-chamber in the same manner as given in the previous chapter. A loose pledget of cotton saturated in an oxyphosphatc cement filling, mixed very thin should be used to seal the cavity. This will not be convenient in many cases and a sandarac varnish dressing may be placed over the cavity. It is better not to seal this cavity with gutta-percha stopping, because of the difficulty in avoiding pressure and forcing the remedy through the canals. Such an accident will cause a very painful toothache for which nothing can be done, except to force warm antiseptic water into the chamber, in the hopes of diluting the drugs. However, it will generally not ache more than half an hour.

This treatment will be sufficient for three or four days, and if the patient requires further treatment the dressing can be removed and in the same manner the tooth prepared for re-dressing, as above. The canals may now be cleaned with a small broach and the treatment again sealed, this time with the gutta-percha stopping. Smooth this with a pledget of cotton saturated in chloroform.

Dr. Buckley is responsible for the perfection of this excellent cresol and formaldehyde treatment, the chemistry of which makes it the rational treatment: The gases ammonia and hydrogen sulphid of putrescent pulp uniting with formaldehyde, urotropin and methyl alcohol and sulphur, are formed. Basic ptomaines, unite with formaldehyde forming inodorous compounds. The cresol (tricresol) is a disinfectant and saponifies the fats. This treatment is used almost universally by dentists and has eliminated to a very great extent the older and inefficient methods of treating this condition.

Non-septic Pericementitis

In the emergency treatment of this condition, the drug irritants which have been used in the pulp extirpation, devitalization and preparation for root filling will have had their effect and this cannot be removed, so relief must be administered. Mechanical irritants, however, such as ill-fitting plates, crowns, bridges, fillings, etc. (except rootcanal fillings), can be removed. It is ill advised for any except the dental surgeon to attempt to remove a rootcanal filling. Crowns or fillings that are left too high may be ground down to relieve the condition.

Immediate relief must be accomplished by the application of drugs and remedies. When a tooth is very sore and has been diagnosed as non-septic pericementitis, one of the ways to relieve it temporarily is to place a silk dental floss around it and slightly pull from the socket. The slight pulling alters the tension in the peridental membrane. It is then a matter of counter-irritation. Wipe the gums as dry as possible around the tooth. Take a pledget of cotton soaked in tincture of iodine tincture of aconite, and chloroform, equal parts, and paint this dry surface, holding the lips and cheeks away until the evaporation ensues. Blowing the surface with a chip blower also adds to the effect.

The patient may be given a small amount of this mixture to paint over the parts, and carefully instructed as to the quantity necessary, etc. Another counter-irritant recommended by Buckley for this is a split raisin, first soaked in hot water and dusted with red pepper, applied to the gums over the tooth. Another remedy for the patient to use is the holding of water, as hot as can be borne, around the tooth. A foot bath, the patient holding his feet for fifteen or thirty minutes, in very hot water, is an excellent remedy.

Chapter Nine - Treatment of Abscess

Acute Alveolar Abscess. — A knowledge of the pathology is more necessary in treating this condition than any other we find. The treatment of acute alveolar abscesses should be abortive in the first stage of the inflammation and pus formation, and in the second stage up to the time the pus perforates through the alveolar process.

The local treatment is to flush clean and sterilize the patient's mouth with the washes advised before; clean and dry the part and place the cotton rolls as previously described. Enlarge the cavity in the tooth until the pulpchamber is opened and with the excavator remove the debris in this part until the root canals can be entered. Take a broach and enter these canals (Fig. 24).

Spontaneous relief from the pain will be noticed when the pus begins to make its appearance into the cavity. An astonishing amount of pus frequently exudes from the apex, five or six drops at a time rushing from the canal. Let this continue to drain. At the first sitting, place a pledget of cotton, saturated in formalin and cresol solution (the excess being removed by touching to a towel) in the bottom of the cavity; cover this with a loose dressing of cotton, soaked in sandarac varnish or vaseline.

At this stage a good counter-irritant may be placed over the gums around the apex (tincture, of iodine, tincture of aconite and chloroform, as given in the preceding chapters). The abortive treatment should be instituted for this stage, a good saline cathartic, as Epsom's salts, or magnesium citrate will prevent an accumulation of blood in the part. An excellent alterative can be given, viz., [1]

R. Potassii iodii..6 gms.
Syrupus sarsaparilla comp...................................90 c.c.
Sig. — Take a teaspoonful in water after meals.

In most cases the pain will subside after the tooth has been treated and the pus evacuated from the cavity, but when the patient is nervous and has lost sleep a good drug to be administered is acetanilid, which may be given in the following form: [2]

R. Pulveris acetanalidum comp............................0.5 gm.
Syrupus simplex..15.0 c.c.
Spiritus frumentii...q. s. ad 90.0 c.c.
Sig. — Take half at once and remainder in two hours if necessary.

When it has been decided that pus has formed and is external to the alveolar process, which can be determined by pressing the finger gently over the part, the treatment of the tooth proper should be the same and the abortive treatment will be altered by the judgment of its necessity. The counter-irritation should not be applied to this outer surface, under any circumstances, at this time, for fear of driving the pus toward the inner wall and into the Antrum of Highmore. Take a lancet, lift the lips and hold clear of the operation, touch the point of the abscess with phenol on the instru-

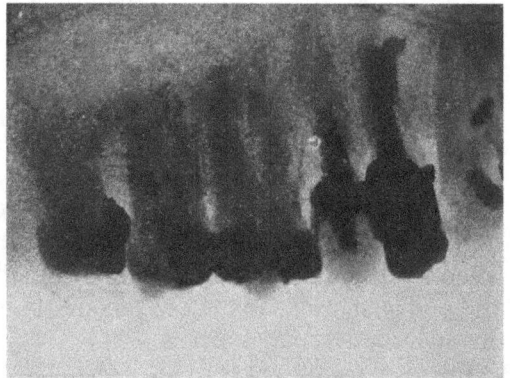

Fig. 25. — Chronic den to-alveolar abscess, with perforation of the root and subsequent forcing of septic matter with gutta-percha through the opening. Three years' duration. Radiograph. — *(Author's practice.)*

40

ment and then force the bistory into the tissue and force it deep, until it touches the alveolar process plate; move it around in the region until the end finds the point of perforation. When this has been drained and all the pus is forced out that can be at this sitting, take a small bundle of cotton fibers, roll very tight, dip in phenol and with a pair of tweezers force to the bottom of the tract and remove. This will take the soreness out of the tissue and cauterize the opening for subsequent escape of pus. The patient should be directed to wash his mouth frequently with one of the washes given before and holding some of the solution in his mouth, to gently massage the swollen part of the face.

The practice of painting the swollen surfaces outside the face with tincture of iodine is good, but it is unsightly and the swelling will generally go down in twenty-four to forty-eight hours after the first treatment. The old method of poulticing on the outside of the face is absolutely uncalled for and criminal.

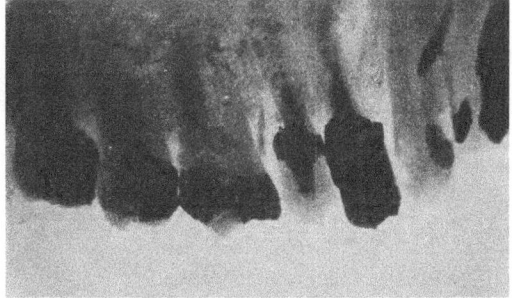

Fig. 26.— Radiograph of case, one week after operation and filling pocket with bismuth paste. — (Author's practice.)

Chronic Alveolar Abscesses

Chronic abscesses, without sinus: The chronic abscesses are, unfortunately for the patient, not so painful and therefore demanding emergency treatment.

The treatment of the chronic abscesses, without fistula is different somewhat from the procedure in the acute abscess, in that the apical opening is entered freely and the contents of the socket stirred to forcible expulsion. The same method of sterilizing the mouth and the use of the cotton rolls and opening the cavity will be followed in this case.

When the canal is opened, there is already a pus sac at the apex

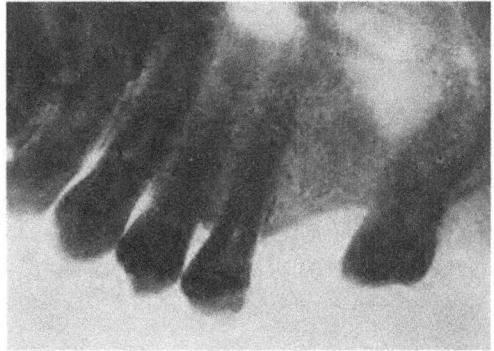

Fig. 27. — Chronic abscess, upper right bicuspid. — (Author's practice.)

and the broach may be forced through into it. Pressure may be applied over this apical part and the pus forced through the canals. These are now cleaned and a loose pledget of cotton, dipped into phenol, placed in the cavity and covered with vaselined cotton. The next sitting, the cotton will be removed

41

and will probably be saturated with pus, which has formed since the first sitting. Drain again, as before and then place a pledget of cotton saturated with the formalin and cresol solution into these canals and seal as tightly as possible, with sandarac varnish or gutta-percha stopping. Remove and re-place this treatment in two or three days, if further attention is demanded.

Chronic abscesses may present for emergency treatment, which are the result of septic matter being forced through a perforated root, as Fig. 25. In the treatment of this case, an opening for drainage was made through the alveolar process, to the point where the foreign substance protruded, this smoothed down and the pari Hushed out and filled with bismuth paste. The second picture, Fig. 26, was taken one week after the operation.

Chronic Alveolar Abscess with Fistula

The treatment of chronic alveolar abscesses with fistula is one which will not generally demand an urgent emergency treatment, because the opening is present and the continual drain eliminates the pain. When one of these abscesses is seen to be drain-ing on the outer surface of the face, an emergency is certainly consid-ered to exist.

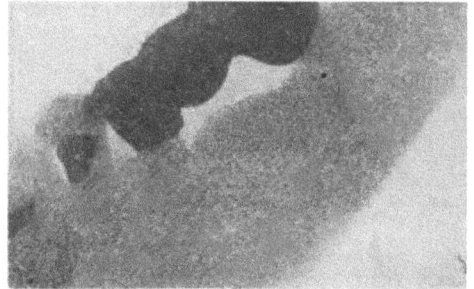

The extraction of a tooth which has a tract opening on the face should be delayed until the scar is healed over. This may be accom-plished by opening the tract inside the mouth, severing it between the point that is bound down and the

Fig. 28. — Chronic dento-alveolar abscess, lower right, third molar. Radiograph. — *(Author's practice.)*

exit through the alveolar process on the inside and turning the drain into the oral cavity. Wait until the outer severed portion of the tract and scar are healed and filled in, and then extract or treat as desired.

The question of extracting teeth when there is an abscess swelling in the mouth is a doubtful one, but the writer believes that this should not be con-sidered dangerous or wrong, as the pus in the abscess will drain readily and he does not believe a secondary infection occurs if the mouth is properly treated and cleaned.

The aim in treating chronic alveolar abscesses with fistula, is to irrigate the tract from the opening in the cavity and the root canals, by forcing a light an-tiseptic bland solution through to the external opening and then place a dressing of formo-cresol solution in the canals for a day or two. The dental surgeon will burn this tract to its extremity with phenosulphuric acid or phenol and fill the root canals. The emergency treatment is to give relief and prevent any complications by making a good-sized opening of the fistula for the drain of the pus and placing a pledget of cotton, rolled on a broach into the canals, and to endeavor to hermetically seal the cavity.

To apply cotton in this way, hold a few fibers of cotton between the thumb and finger of the left hand, place the end of the broach in this and twist, holding the ends of the cotton with the same finger of the right hand. Dip it in the solution, place in the canal and holding the cotton in place with the beaks of a pair of dressing pliers on either side, withdraw the broach.

This will be sufficient to meet the demands of emergency treatment, in chronic cases, the completion of which should not be delayed until a dental surgeon is available.

[1] Buckley.   [2] Harlan lectures.

Chapter Ten - Neuralgia

When the condition present is evidently not one described in the chapter on dental pain and a cure cannot be affected by the methods given for affected teeth, we look to a solution of the dilemma in Neuralgia.

Neuralgia (Nerve Pain)

Neuralgia is a manifestation of the disorder produced by overexcitation of the sensory nerves or by perverted function. Reflex pain is a pain experienced at some point other than that of its origin. Neuralgia is described as a stinging, severe, paroxysmal pain along the course or part of the course of a nerve and in the area of its distribution. Neuralgia occurs in many organs and parts of the body and except for those reflected from dental sources will be treated by the general practitioner.

The dental operator is called upon to treat chiefly those which appear in the region of distribution or along the course of the fifth cranial nerve. These are called tri-facial, facial and trigeminal neuralgia.

Marshall [1] gives a very comprehensive and complete idea of causes of neuralgia, in the following.

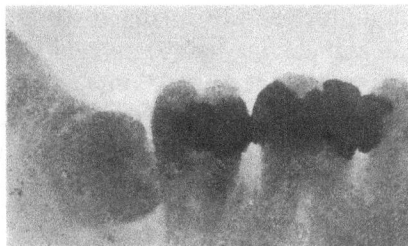

Fig. 29. — Impacted third molar. A hidden cause of facial neuralgia. Radiograph. — *(Author's practice.)*

"The conditions which are productive of neuralgia are many and varied and consist chiefly of diseases which lower the vital powers of the system, such as anemia, or those which interfere with such functions as the circulation, respiration, digestion, assimilation, secretion and elimination; the presence in the system of abnormal substances as in gout, rheumatism, diabetes, malaria, nephritis, chronic pyemia, syphilis and metallic poisoning, local conditions which cause reflex peripheral irritation, such as diseases of the teeth, eye, ears, stomach, uterus and ovaries; chronic inflammation of the nerve or its sheath, pressure from abnormal growths, within the bony canal through which the nerve trunk passes, or pressure from tumors and localized anemia or congestion of nerves or nerve centers."

Facial Neuralgia for consideration in this chapter will be divided into two classes: those arising from dental sources and those arising from other than dental sources. In the first class we find:

Exposed dentine around the necks of the teeth, as a result of abrasion, neuralgic pains may be produced by merely touching these surfaces with an instrument, or even with the finger nail.

Pulpitis. — The pain may be referred to another part or area than its origin.

Pulp nodules, or pulp stones and secondary dentine affections outnumber all other conditions as causes.

Pericementitis. — Generally the pain is located over the affected tooth, yet it may not be and the pain be referred from this point.

Cementosis. — This is one of the more common causes of facial neuralgia, because of the pressure of the growth against the nerve trunk or sheath.

Deposits. — Calcic deposits on the roots of teeth.

Impacted Teeth. — Maleruption of the lower third molars is the most frequent example of neuralgia from this source because of its anatomical relation with the inferior dental nerve which courses the inner part of the maxillary bone. Fig. 29 shows a case of Neuralgia, which ceased upon extraction. From this source, however, the pain will generally be localized in the part.

Burchard and Inglis state that "an equivalent of impaction in which dental irritation may be the source of reflex neuralgia, is when the teeth are crowded or jammed into arches too small for their accommodation." Deafness, suppurative otitis media, disturbances of the eye, temporary blindness, ovarian and uterine neuralgia, sciatica, pains in the knee, toes, fingers, have been traced to dental irritation.

Those cases which present neuralgia from other than dental sources are just the opposite of the above, the pain definitely located or indefinitely located in a normal tooth referred from some other source.

The condition in which this occurs are malaria, gout, syphilis, diseases of the brain, kidneys, uterus, bladder, disorders in pregnancy, diseases of the fifth cranial nerve, constipation and la-grippe.

The paramount point in neuralgia is to find the cause and make the proper diagnosis. The X-ray in many cases, is the only method by which we may discover an irritating cause.

The cause found, the treatment is to remove it and should it be a tooth, diagnose the condition and treatment for this as described in previous chapters. Do not extract the tooth unless deemed absolutely necessary for relief.

Local application of drugs which act upon the sensory nerve ending will be used and Buckley's dental liniment which follows, will give excellent results.

R. Mentholis...1.3 gms.
Chloroform...6.0 c.c.
Tinct. Aconite...30.0 c.c.
Sig. — Paint over the area affected.

Another liniment recommended by Buckley:

R. Mentholis...2.0 gms.
Alcoholis,
Aetheris...āā 24.00 c.c.
Chloroformi...90.00 c.c.

Sig. — Apply by vigorous rubbing or massage over the area of distribution of the affected nerves or along its course.

In many cases where pain in the upper teeth is caused by abscessed teeth or affections of the peridental membrane, the following may be used with wonderful results, stopping the pain almost instantly. [2]

R. Alcoholis...
Aquae...āā 30.00 c.c.
Sig. — Use as a spray well back in the nostril of the side affected. Repeat as often as necessary.

When general medicinal treatment is demanded for correction of the constitutional disorder or alteration of treatment necessary, the physician in charge will make these changes. Dentists have kept patients suffering for some unnecessary length of time when searching for a cause in the mouth when it was a general or constitutional condition, and doctors, just the same, have treated patients for months without result, until the dentist removed or treated the offending teeth.

While an operator is searching for a hidden cause it is his duty to administer hypnotic or general anodyne or analgesic and the prescriptions of some of the best in writer's experience follow:

R. Pulveris acetanilidum comp.........gr. xx (1.3 gms.)

Fiat chartulae no. iv. Sig. — Take one powder every hour until two or three are taken, if not relieved after two hours, take the remaining one or two.

The use of phenacetine is very good in these cases, combined with codeine sulphate or salophen.

R. Acetaphenacetinae,
Salophen...āā gr. xx (1.3 gms.)

Codienae sulphatis..............................gr. i (0.6 gms.)
Fiat chartulae no. iv.
Sig.— Take one powder every two hours.

Neuralgia cases will be very materially aided by the following prescription which is simple and efficient.

R. Acetanilidum.................................gr. vii (0.5 gms.)
Syrupi simplex.....................................fl℈ss (15.0 c.c.)
Spiritus frumentii qs. ad. fl℥ (90 c.c.)
Sig. — Take one-half at once and the remainder in two hours.

When these remedies will not suffice and the patient is in such a condition to justify the last resort, the use of morphine will meet the demand. Prescription should not be given. A dose of 1/8 gr. (0.008 gm.) may be given by the stomach, repeated in one-half or one hour and the patient given one more tablet to take at home if necessary. This is the conservative amount that the patient should take in emergency cases. The patient should be given a good cathartic, always; and If the conditions persist a hot foot bath, as advised before, will aid in the relief.

[1] "Injuries and Surgical Diseases of the Face, Mouth and Jaws."
[2] Buckley.

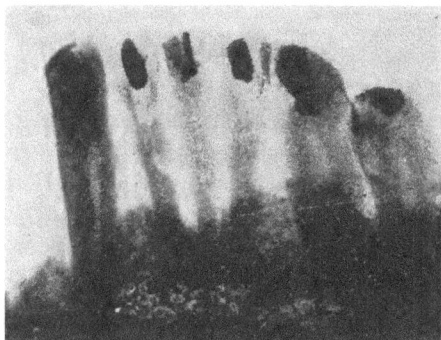

Fig. 30. — Pyorrhea alveolaris. Radiograph. — *(Author's practice.)*

Chapter Eleven - Pyorrhea Alveolaris

This is an acute or chronic inflammatory process which includes the following features:

A molecular necrosis of the peridental membrane (organ of attachment of the tooth in the socket). See Fig. 15, Chapter V.

Atrophy of the alveolar walls.

Hyperemia of the gums.

Pus (generally at some stage) oozing out from around the necks of the teeth.

Calcic deposits on the roots of the teeth. Looseness and falling out of the teeth.

This disease is as old as man; people of all races, all stations and climates and time and modes of life have suffered from it.

It has been studied exhaustively since the year 1746 when Fauchard [1] published a description of it and from that time to this, many able men have occupied their time and thoughts seeking satisfactory explanation of its phenomena.

It is the most named disease in medical science. Each writer having observed some particular symptom, which was paramount in his observation, made a title which conveyed his idea.

The various titles are therefore descriptive of symptoms or stages of this condition. Among the more common titles which are or have been in use are: Pyorrhea alveolaris, interstitial gingivitis, Riggs disease, calcic inflammation, hematogenic calcic pericementitis, gouty pericementitis. There are practically two schools regarding this condition, one contending a *local* and the other a *general constitutional etiology.*

The local adherents cling to the following conditions as the causative elements; viz., subgingival deposits of calculi, acute inflammation of the mucous membrane, catarrhal conditions, germs, stomatitis, irregular teeth, malocclusion, non-occlusion and uncleanliness.

Those who maintain the general or constitutional etiology, ascribe it to general condition of health, heredity, gouty diathesis, excessive lime salt secretions, meat eating, nervous exhaustion, scorbutus, environment and uric acid. Burchard describes the course of the disease as three stages: i. Tooth induration; 2. erosion by chemical solution of the crowns of the teeth; 3. loss of retaining structures of the teeth.

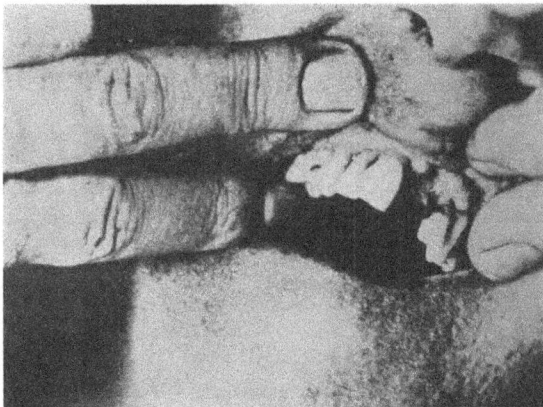

Fig. 31. — Pyorrhea alveolaris, left central incisor, exfoliated.

The reader should consult the chart, Fig. 15, Chapter V, for the relative position of the structures, especially the alveolar sockets, the pericementum and gum tissues.

Regarding the local causes, when there is an excess of salts in the blood and these are not eliminated, it is readily seen that such an ideal place as the free margins of the gums, becomes a seat of deposition. Acute inflammation follows and extends over the gum tissue which becomes turgid and spongy. It then attacks the delicate peridental membrane, which is defenseless by reason of its location, functions, etc. This is the most vulnerable point for this process and for the development of bacteria, and eventually of pus.

The blood-vessels pass in a plexus from the periosteum to the peridental membrane, and under normal conditions remove the calcium salts. It will readily be seen, however, that under the perverted condition of irritation and disturbed

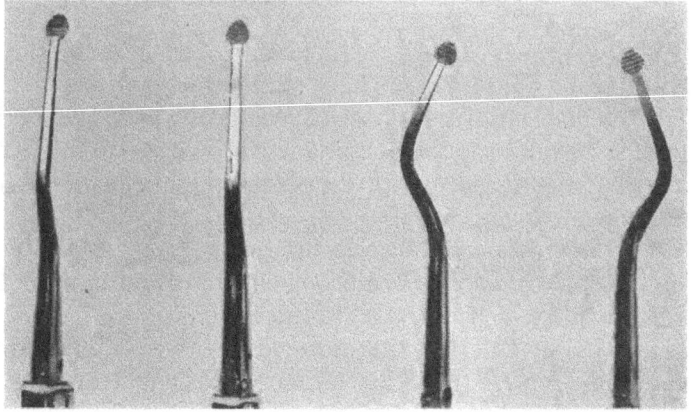

Fig. 32. Instruments used in emergency treatment of pyorrhea alveolaris.

nutrition, this function will be hindered and the deposition of salts will occur instead of their removal. Irregular teeth, malocclusion, and non-occlusion add to this possibility by improper mastication and interrupted functions of the teeth, which should maintain a healthy condition. Inflammation will result from mechanical and chemical causes and as this proceeds infection is inevitable, as the oral cavity constantly harbors disease-producing organisms.

The specific organisms causing the infection and the pus formation have not been isolated and the various forms found have not been sufficient to produce the disease by inoculation with single strains.

Talbot says, "the pathogenic conception adopted anent interstitial gingivitis is that the disorder is a local inflammatory condition of the gums, etc." [2]

The general or constitutional causes are much discussed and disputed conditions. There can be no doubt that with a disrupted condition of health, we will have degenerative conditions of the various organs and an abnormal amount of salts present and failure in proper elimination increases the probability of their effect on this disease.

Heredity is claimed to exert an exceptionally large influence in some cases.

The gouty diathesis is the form which has been the subject of so much discussion.

However, when a case persists and does not yield to local treatment and the institution of constitutional treatment for the gout is accompanied by great improvement in the pyorrhea we are prone to believe that this is a cause of the condition under discuss on.

The principal point, which this brings out is that of improper elimination and irritation of uric acid, urates and calcium salts, in the deposition next to the peridental membrane. Pierce believes this to be the local manifestation of the gouty diathesis. [3]

Talbot, however, after various and exhaustive experimentation has found such a small percentage of pyorrhea teeth deposits to contain uric acid and urates that he has come to the conclusion that "uric acid when it acts at all, acts as a local irritant. The general circulation, carrying an excess of salts as in excessive lime salt secretion, deposits it through the process spoken of above, when it becomes a local irritant.

Nervous exhaustion is considered for the effects that follow in the structure and the reduction in tone of the immediate organs of supply. Uric acid is given as a result in gouty pericementitis. Its presence and' irritation is one of the main points, in the class considered to be of constitutional etiology.

It is the aim of the writer to present to the reader only an outline of the disease, as it will be

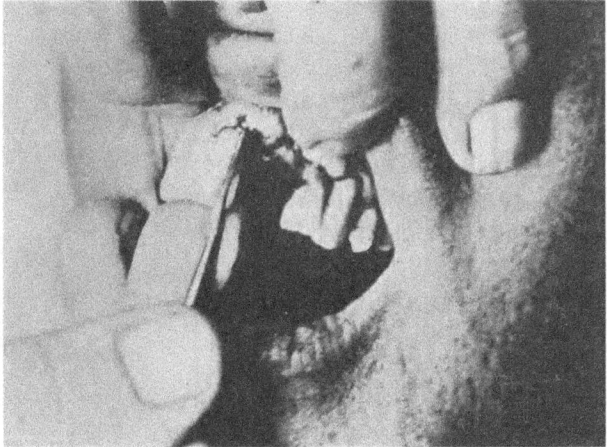

Fig. 33. — Pyorrhea alveolaris, showing instrument, angle and fingers used in scaling tartar.

presented for diagnosis and enough of the ideas of the energetic men who have contributed so much toward clearing up the baffling conditions, to make it intelligently understood.

There is not space in this work to deal otherwise with this condition.

The diagnosis of pyorrhea alveolaris will be by sight and touch. The gums are generally red, turgid and congested. Pressure will bring a show of pus. Pain in the alveolar sockets is not usually experienced. This point is the unfortunate part in the disease, because an unobserving patient will not know of its existence. Hard, black, brown or" yellow calculus will be found attached to the sides of the roots and the gum tissue will at times cover this. A pus-pocket may exist along the side of the root unobserved, except that the tract or the seepage will be noticed at the gum margins. An offensive odor attends the progress of the disease, especially in unhygienic mouths. The diagnosis can be confounded with a few other conditions, such as gingivitis, stomatitis, mercurial ptyalism, impacted teeth, or effects of ill-fitting dentures. It makes its appearance generally between thirty-five and fifty years of age, with symptoms practically the same as acute non-septic pericementitis. The color of the gums is deep red or purple, over the ends of the roots of the teeth affected. Constitutional conditions which may cause pyorrhea and upon which diagnostic symptoms may depend will be gleaned from the history.

Treatment

The treatment of pyorrhea alveolaris in emergency cases is to give relief from pain and save teeth. The teeth frequently are very loose and appear to have little attachment, but after the first treatment and institution of prophylaxis, they will tighten to a surprising amount. Extraction in chronic cases is practised where the absorption of the peridental membrane and process has gone beyond repair, but in the first-aid treatment that procedure should seldom be resorted to. Acute pains of the abscess variety will cause the patient to seek relief; and in this, temporary treatment will do a great deal more than might be supposed. The patient will present with severe pains around the roots of the affected teeth. The gums will be purplish and swollen; pressure on the teeth will respond as in abscesses. The hyperemia and

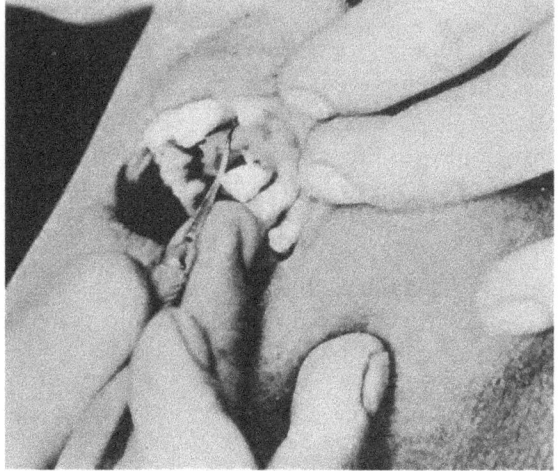

Fig. 34. — Pyorrhea alveolaris instrumentation.

the pain of the gums will be a diagnostic sign. There will generally be deposit on the roots under the gums; and the teeth may be somewhat loose. It is our duty to relieve this patient without delay. There is no satisfaction in telling him that he has pyorrhea alveolaris and cannot be cured; and we cannot be barbarous enough to extract the teeth affected, especially at this sitting.

Wash the mouth with one of the solutions given before and use a syringe to Hush out the spaces as previously stated, the solutions should be hot. As in all diseases the first rational step is to remove the cause.

If the condition has a constitutional basis, it will be reduced through systemic channels. The following treatment will be necessary in this as it will in the local condition, as the local effect must be repaired.

Fig. 32 shows four pyorrhea instruments or files, which the writer believes will be sufficient to treat emergency cases. The pyorrhea specialist uses from twelve to one hundred instruments for the treatment of this condition; including every angle and edge to suit conditions and manner of operation in removal of tartar. These four instruments will be used as shown in Figs. 33 and 34, to enter under the free margins of the gums and file down or cut away the hard deposits. In doing this care must be taken to follow the sides of the teeth and enter through the tracts leading to the pockets.

50

Remove all the hard deposits found and flush out the edges of the pockets with an ordinary mouth syringe and a warm solution. The gums will bleed freely and will appear to be very badly injured, but when these pockets have been scaled and the gums massaged the relief given by the hemorrhage will be apparent.

The practice of using orange wood sticks or any other methods of placing strong acids in these sockets in emergency treatment or permanent treatment is condemned. A surgeon does not apply acids to a fractured joint as a treatment under any circumstances, septic or aseptic, since necrosis would result. The same reasoning applies in this condition. We want to make tissue grow, not destroy it, and nature should be given an unhampered opportunity. We should treat these cases with the idea of getting rid of the tartar, the pus and the excess blood and then use the following remedy which will prevent the germs of the oral cavity from entering and adding to the infection.

Hartzell [4] has given us the remedy of painting the gum margins with tincture of iodine and creosote and following this with glycerite of tannin, which will be seen to be a powerful astringent and anodyne, sealing the edges of the gums around the necks of the teeth.

Place cotton rolls on the outside of the gums on the upper jaw, and on either side on the lower. Being positive that the pus and tartar have been removed, take a small pledget of cotton, saturated in the tincture of iodine and creosote, and paint around the gum margins and necks of the teeth. Take another pledget and sear over these with the glycerite of tannin. This should be left for twenty-four hours and the patient instructed not to brush his teeth. However, the patient should be instructed to use the toothbrush the next day. A softer brush than medium, should never be used, the hard bristles should usually be advised. Brushing the gums with soft brushes does not give them the exercise and friction necessary to reduce them, when soft and spongy, to a hard healthy condition.

The patient should be instructed to massage the gums with the finger, which is a difficult process in some parts of the mouth. The writer advises that the patient hold a small amount of a warm astringent solution in the mouth and with the cotton rolls shown in Fig. 19 on the finger, go all around the gums. The patient should be instructed to brush his teeth as directed in Chapter II.

The cause being considered constitutional and the condition in the mouth as a local manifestation, the above treatment should be applied and the patient given a good cathartic, advised to drink a large quantity of water and abstain from the eating of foods which carry much lime salts.

Constitutional treatment will be directed by the surgeon.

[1] "The American Text-book on Operative Dentistry."
[2] "Interstitial Gingivitis."
[3] "American Text-book of Operative Dentistry."
[4] "Dental Cosmos," 1913, p. 1094.

Chapter Twelve - Fractures and Dislocations of the Jaws and Their Treatment

The word fracture means the breaking of a bone or cartilage.

Stimson gives the following classification of the various kinds of fractures, with which are given subdivisions under each head.

1. Incomplete Fractures.
2. Complete Fractures.
3. Multiple Fractures.
4. Compound Fractures.
5. Gunshot Fractures.

The causes of the fractures of the bones of the face are many and varied. The superior maxillary bone is not prone to fracture because of its position and protection by the various processes. Fractures of the bones are always produced by direct violence and present variance according to their etiology. The various processes are fractured with violent blows, a blow on the cheek may break the malar bone and fracture the anterior border of the antrum, as also a fractured nose may include the nasal process. The alveolar process may be broken up extensively by a blow on the mouth, or in the extraction of teeth such a blow may separate the palatal process from the body of the bone. Stimson quotes a

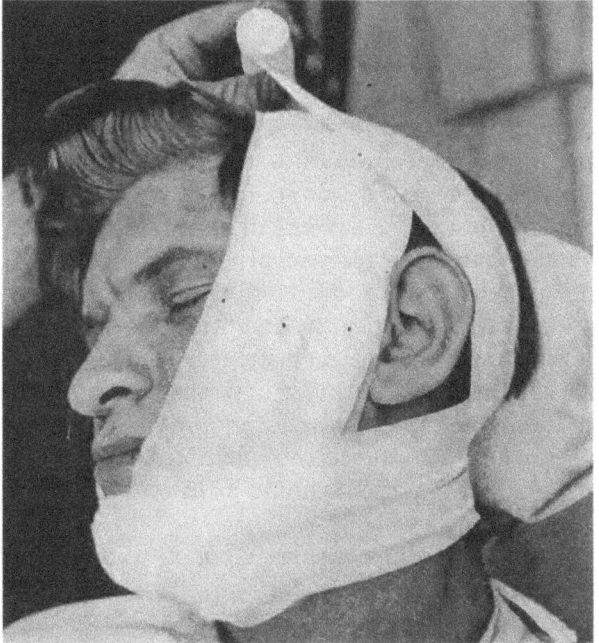

Fig. 35. — Bandaging the jaws together (modified-Barton's). Front view.

case of his practice, in which the face was crushed in an elevator, ... "the nasal bones were separated from the frontal along the suture line, the right malar and zygoma broken; and both superior maxillae displaced downward and backward and separated from each other along the median line of the hard palate." In one case the bones of the face were so movable that they moved up and down when the patient swallowed, as if they were only restrained by the skin. In order to produce these conditions, the extreme violence necessary and the extent of the injury would seem necessarily to involve the cranium, but the reason given for the cranium's immunity, is that the direction of the force is always more or less parallel to the surface of the cranium.

Comminuted (splintered fragments of bone) fractures often occur in gunshot wounds and injuries of all descriptions. The diagnosis of this fracture is comparatively easy and can be made without difficulty because the mouth and external surface afford easy access for manipulation with the fingers. It presents an irregular outline, displacement, mobility and crepitus.

These cases are treated by placing the parts in proper relation and retaining them. The method advised in this chapter is that of fixation of the upper to the lower jaw by the process of wiring the teeth.

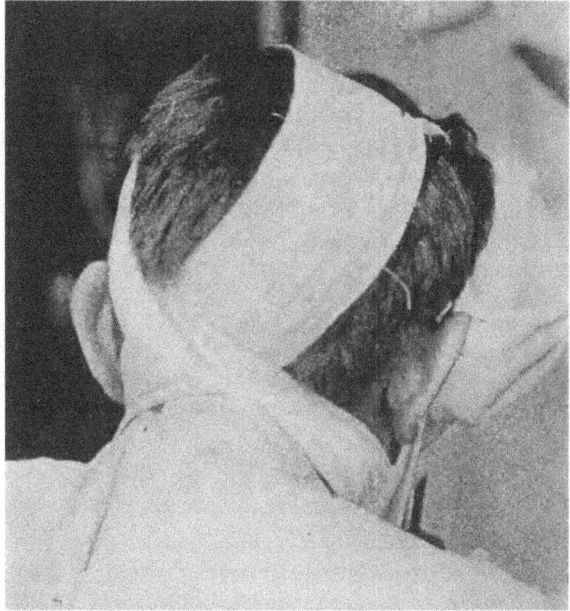

Fig. 36. — Rear view of Fig. 35.

In the fracture of the alveolar process, place the fragments of bone in proper position and the teeth in their sockets and fix by wiring or apply splints made of gutta-percha over the cutting edges of the teeth and parts.

Loose teeth should be replaced in the sockets, no matter how loose they appear to be in the fracture, as they will eventually tighten in place. Extraction endangers because of possible removal of the part or parts of bone.

Fractures of the Inferior Maxilla

This fracture is more common and important from the dental operator's standpoint as injuries of the upper face will usually be dealt with by the surgeon.

The technical knowledge of the relationship of the jaws and the occlusion of the teeth, together with the manipulation of these parts brings the operation of the inferior maxilla under the dentist's care.

Fractures of this bone generally occur in patients between the ages of twenty and thirty. It is the most commonly fractured bone of the face by rea-

53

son of its location and function. Its fracture is much more common in men than in women.

Incomplete fractures of the mandible are those which only include the alveolar process or some part of the border of the bone. Complete fractures are those in which the fracture extends through the entire bone, divided or classified by the direction of the fracture as oblique, longitudinal, transverse, etc., and comminuted.

Compound fractures are those in which the membrane covering the bone is broken or cut. They present an open wound.

Gunshot fractures are as the name implies.

In the extraction of teeth, in blows, falls or any external violence against the teeth or face, the alveolar process is very liable to be broken, as is also a part of the border.

The writer has recently had a case of fracture of the mandible, in which the external plate of the alveolar process was fractured from the right to the left cuspid tooth with a small triangular fragment broken from the body of the bone. His history showed fracture seven years before. There had been continual drain from the lower central incisors, which moreover were affected with pyorrhea alveolaris. The displaced alveolar plate became firm, but the fragment of the body of the bone was removed because of necrosis, Figs. 37 and 38, and the two central incisors were later extracted.

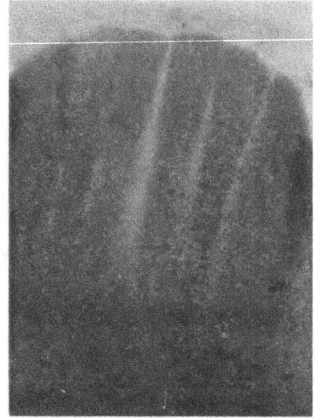

Fig. 37. — Fracture. Case 1 — Maxillary process, involving border of body of maxillary bone. Radiograph. — *(Author's practice.)*

Complete fractures occur more frequently in the anterior portion of the bone. Stimson states that of 75 single ones of these, the fractures occupied the median line in 25, the region of the anterior in 22, that of the back teeth in 15, behind the teeth in 8 and in the condyloid process in 5."

In the writer's experience the majority of cases have been multiple fractures, mostly double. This condition has been obtained probably by reason of the difficulties in these cases, the necessity of dental technic, affording the opportunity in consultation. The fracture of the body of the bone generally has a vertical direction; in the ramus, it is usually oblique.

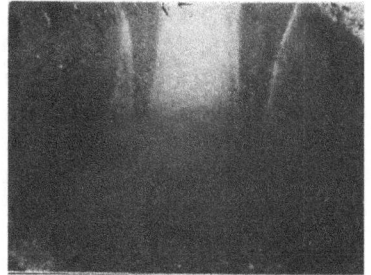

Fig. 38. — Case 1, one month after removal of sequestra and teeth, process firmly re-attached. Radiograph. — *(Author's practice.)*

The fractures through the symphysis or the vicinity of the anterior teeth do not show great displacement, part of the lines of occlusion of the teeth being correct, however, a slight separation of the teeth in the respective fragments will generally be noted. Posterior to the cuspid teeth, the fracture will be more easily noted, the abnormal occlusion being prominent because of the action of the masseter and pterygoid muscles.

In a case in the writer's practice a simple fracture through the symphysis was not noticed for three weeks after the accident, when inability to masticate brought the patient for treatment. In shooting a rifle, the rebound caused the stock to come forcibly in contact with the point of the chin and a vertical fracture resulted.

Another case of compound fracture presented. A patient while under the influence of alcohol was struck on the point of the chin, from the right side and neglected treatment for several days. Examination showed a fracture through the body of the bone at the left of the lower left lateral incisor, one through the socket of the right cuspid and one anterior to the second

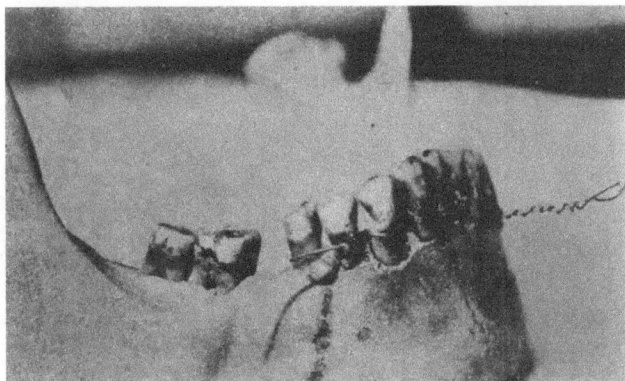

Fig. 39. — Dr. O. T. Oliver's method of wiring across the fracture. Pencil mark representing fracture.

molar, the first molar being absent. The mouth was foul and infected, the patient at the time had various venereal diseases. The anterior fragment was drawn directly back into the mouth, the teeth pointing almost toward the tongue, the other fragment was drawn in also, the anterior part overlapping the former, the posterior portion was in good position.

In another case, the patient received a blow on the point of the chin with a stool, with fracture through the symphysis, and between the second bicuspid and first molar. Patient had failed to report and infection followed, the jaw had been lanced on the outer surface and drained. The parts were not in very bad alignment and were painful only upon movement. A large amount of necrosis followed in this

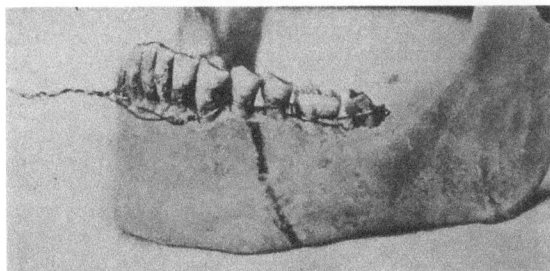

Fig. 40.— Method of lacing teeth and wiring across the fracture, wires loosely applied for photographic clearness.]

case, with resultant removal of sequestra.

Many cases of abscess opening into the mouth are associated with small fragments of bone, these are exfoliations or splinters and must be removed.

The diagnosis of fractures of the inferior maxilla is comparatively simple, as the observation of the parts and manipulations will show abnormal mobility, crepitus, displacement and pain.

Treatment

There are many and varied means of treating these cases; and as is true of all conditions, many which answer, but are not sufficient. The treatment of the mouth should be taken first and the hot solution of one of the mouth washes used to flush it out. The use of a swab of cotton to go gently over all the teeth and get the field as clean as possible makes the patient grateful, the working in the cavity more pleasant and safer. The class and extent of the fracture should be determined and the method of retaining selected.

In edentulous jaws, where there is no occlusion of the teeth to determine the proper placing of

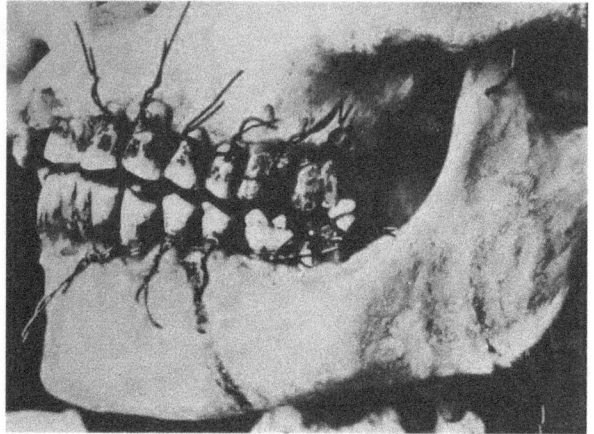

Fig. 41. — Wires in place on the teeth previous to reduction and twisting.

the parts; the use of the four-tailed bandage and gutta-percha splints will be found the best method of retention.

A wax mold should be made of the upper and lower jaw and a wax bite secured, plaster casts made and mounted on an articulator, over which warm gutta-percha should be molded, cooled and trimmed to fit the case. Insert in position and apply the bandage using a pad covered by a piece of wet cardboard under the chin, Figs. 35 and 36.

The method of wiring

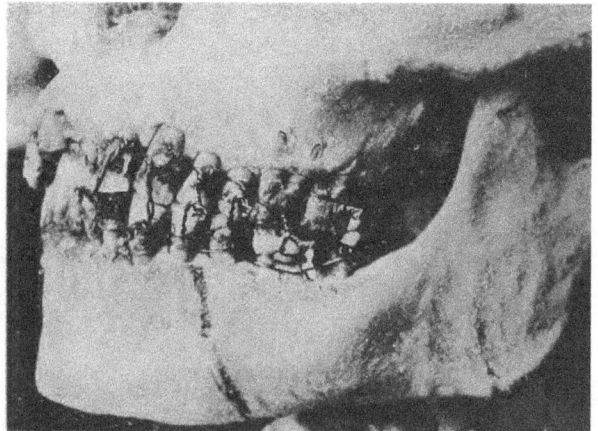

Fig. 42. — Wires twisted showing free end, before bending into spaces between teeth.

the teeth, in the author's opinion, presents the quickest and easiest as well as the most sanitary and surest method of proper retention. The parts of the fracture are brought directly before the eye of the operator, during the entire operation and treatment. In complicated cases, it serves the purpose far better than splints, because of ability to reduce gradually or separate the jaws without disturbing the union. There is no method whereby control from mobility can be secured as with the wiring process.

In the first case cited an X-ray plate was made, Fig. 37, which showed there was not a complete fracture, the lower teeth were tied together in the sockets and an alignment wire placed over the entire lower set, by inter-lacing with twenty gauge wire. The jaws were fastened together for ten days. The wound was dressed and packed with gauze, dipped in iodoform, orthoform and campho-phcnique paste. The case was painful and the drain of the pus persisted. Removal of the two central incisors and incision was made over the fragment of bone which was removed and the case was practically cured, Fig. 38.

Robert T. Oliver [1] has given a method of wiring a slightly transverse fracture through the socket distally of the first bicuspid and mental foramen. He uses copper wire, annealed, about 4 inches long, inserts one end through the space between the lateral and canine teeth, burnishes lingually to the canine, pulls through half the length, brings it back through between the

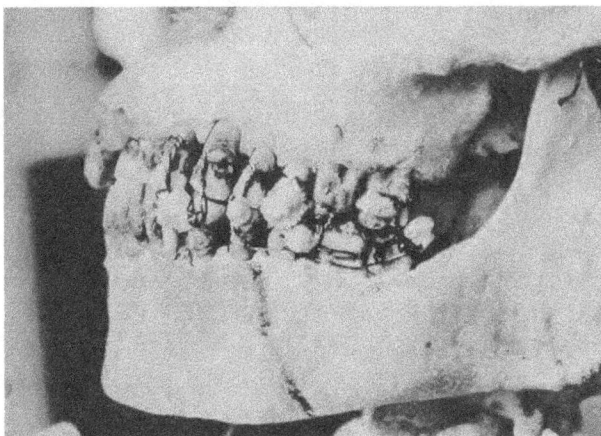

Fig. 42a. — Twisted ends of wires turned in and covered with gutta-percha to protect the lips.

canine and bicuspid, then the other end is inserted between the canine and bicuspid, burnished to the lingual side of the first and second bicuspids, carried back across the fracture, inserted from within through the space between the first molar and second bicuspid, brought forward taut and the ends twisted.

Fig. 40 shows the author's method of reducing by lacing the teeth with a wire about 6 inches long and bringing the cross forward between each tooth except the two adjoining teeth on either side of the fracture, where the wire extends along each side of the two approximating teeth, then to cross again, the cuspid encircled and the ends of the wires twisted at the cuspid tooth.

This process is used in fractured bones to draw together and retain the parts. The teeth of the full upper jaw are wired as follows: Small wires about 2 inches long are placed tightly around the gingival margins under the gums and twisted in the same direction, preferably to the right, on each tooth. The number of the teeth wired in this manner will be determined by the amount of fixation deemed necessary. The lower teeth opposite the uppers are all wired to correspond with the other and the wires turned forward in the mouth. Fig. 41.

The reducing wire is twisted until the parts appear to be together in contact and then the jaws are closed and held by an assistant. Then on the side which is not fractured, twist the wires of opposing teeth until the cusps are almost in proper contact. Fig. 42; the fractured side is then drawn up in the same manner as near as possible. If the parts are swollen or too painful absolute contact will be difficult and in this method it is unnecessary, since the parts can be moved or reduced gradually for seven days.

Place a bandage over the head as shown in Fig. 35, to counteract the muscular contraction which tends to break the wires. A gauze pack covered by a piece of wet cardboard is molded over the skin and this is covered by the bandage, which need only be worn for a few days.

Traction on these fragments is nearly always desired and the wiring process presents full possibilities for the action required. This is the great advantage over all other methods. Dr. Oliver [2] describes an original method of constructing an anchor loop for the alignment wire, of either upper or lowers, by twisting a copper wire around a mandrel thus making a loop, which can be tacked with hard solder and placed at the point desired for application of the traction wire.

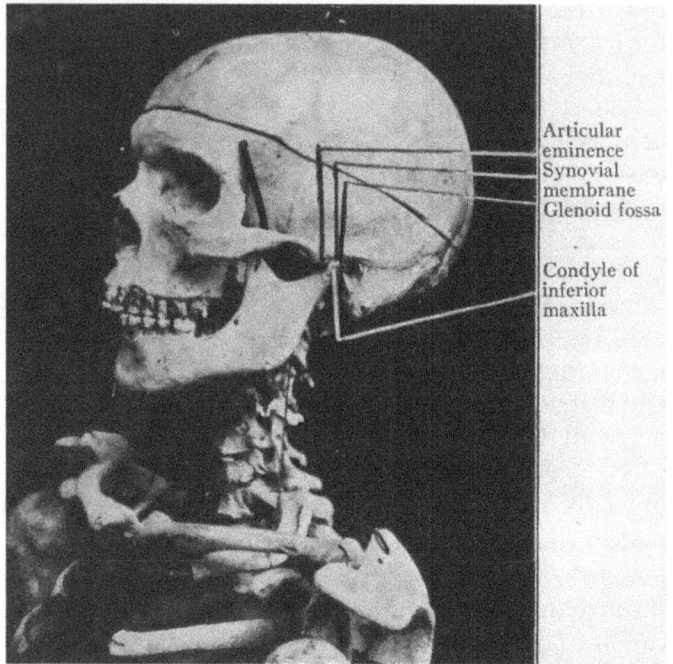

Fig. 43. — **Temporo maxillary articulation.**

There is no necessity for extracting any teeth in this method for feeding purposes as the patient under any circumstances is required to subsist on liquid diet and the entrance of this has sufficient space around the posterior teeth. The patient may also be fed by a tube passed through the nostril.

The wires are cut short and covered with wax or guttapercha, which is changed daily. Fig. 42a. They are brushed with a small brush, syringed out and a good mouth wash advised. Hydrogen peroxide is valuable in the wash for cleaning around the wires.

In cases where union is delayed, with the lower jaw wired to the upper and the alignment wires in place, it is a simple matter to loosen the jaws by untwisting the wires; if it is necessary to incise and scrape the edges of the fracture or remove sequestra or splinters. Where the union of the fragments demands that the wire be placed through the bone, the process is simple Make an incision, through the soft tissue in a line along the body of the bone, separate the soft parts from the bone then with a spear point or cone-shaped drill, make a hole through the process between the teeth on either side of the fracture, being careful to have plenty of structure between the edges of the fracture and the hole. Place a twenty gauge silver wire through the hole, with the free ends on the outside, twist until apposition is secured. Leave this twisted part of the wire about an inch long and if necessary stitch the wound

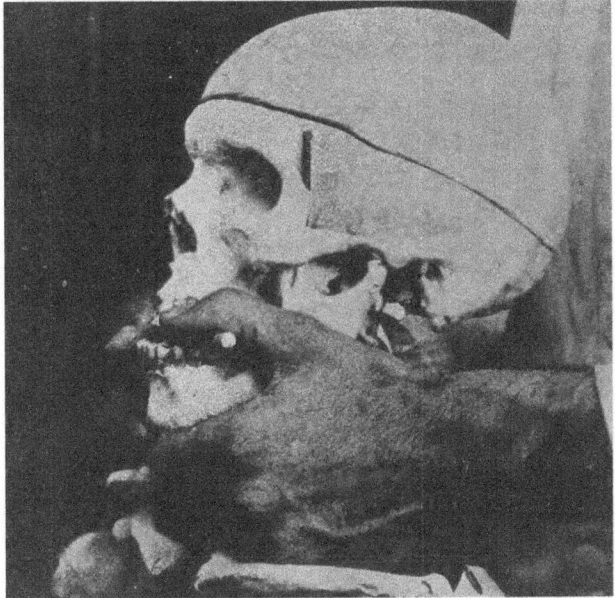

Fig. 44. — Method of reducing dislocated maxilla with use of pencil between the teeth.

on either side, leaving the twisted ends of the wire exposed. When the union is accomplished, clip the posterior portion of the wire beneath the twisted part and carefully remove it by holding the twisted portion in a pair of pliers and pulling forward along the line of the bone.

Cases should heal in from three to six weeks and without deformity or improper occlusion, such as often results where the teeth are hidden from view by the use of splints.

Dislocation of Lower Jaw

There is nothing so distressing to the patient as a dislocation of the lower jaw. A study of the anatomy of the part will show the comparative ease with which the dislocation occurs. It occurs in from 3 to 6 per cent, of all dislocations. Fig. 43 shows the joint in proper relationship with the parts noted.

The glenoid fossa is the socket which, lined with a pad, the synovial membrane, receives the condyle of the inferior maxilla. The articular eminence forms the anterior border of the fossa. In dislocations, the condyle comes forward over this eminence.

Backward and internal or external dislocations are rare, without other complications. The condyle is attached by ligaments, the capsular, internal and external lateral, which are stretched during the dislocation.

Relaxation of these ligaments and contraction of the muscles, violence in the mouth, laughing, shouting, yawning, vomiting and dental extractions, are the most common causes of dislocation, one or both sides may be dislocated.

The symptoms of the condition include a protrusion of the lower teeth, a depression in front of the car and inability of the patient to manipulate the jaw. If unilateral, the chin will point to the opposite side.

The *treatment* is the reduction of the condition which ordinarily in recent cases is not difficult.

Fig. 44 illustrates one method of reduction, after placing a pencil, a small stick or cork between the molar teeth, the operator standing at the patient's back, by upward pressure on the chin forces the condyle down to a level with the articular eminence, a slight pull aided by the action of the muscles, will then be sufficient to snap the jaw into place.

The thumbs of the operator may be bandaged and placed in the mouth, operator in front of patient and pressure made on the molar teeth with an upward force applied under the chin and relocation gained in this manner.

The use of the jaw should be limited for a few days; in severe cases a bandage, as shown above, applied for such time as the operator deems necessary.

[1] "Dental Cosmos," Sept., 1911.   [2] "Dental Cosmos," 1911.

Chapter Thirteen - Dental Extractions

Throughout this book, appeal has been made to save the teeth. When extraction has been decided upon it will be assumed that all the resources of treatment have been exhausted Many writers have made various rules for dentists to follow in deciding to extract, but with all respect to them, the judgment of the operator in each case must decide.

It is impossible to pull certain teeth, which with proper manipulation will yield with comparative ease. The procedure described by the expression that "the patient was dragged all over the office or that the operator pulled with all his strength, etc.," is barbarous and absolutely unnecessary. The erroneous idea given by the words "pulling or drawing teeth' 7 will be eliminated and replaced by the proper words "extracting or removing teeth."

The nervous condition of the patient tends to influence the operator to hurry and there is no operation which demands deliberate and concise actions as does extracting.

Improper methods and ill-applied force cause so many accidents in extraction of teeth that exact knowledge of the structures and their relations is necessary. The accidents include fracturing the jaw or alveolar process, removing parts of the floor of the maxillary sinus, fracturing of other teeth, extraction of the wrong or more than one tooth and in injuries to the tongue and soft tissues. The points given under the extraction of each tooth, will aid in rational extraction.

Failures, accidents and complications occur in extractions and these must be guarded against by a study of the parts, knowledge of the eruption of teeth, care and proper manipulation of instruments and consideration of oral sepsis, during and after operation.

Failures in removing all of the root or roots of teeth occur for various reasons. Some teeth present a ball at the end of the root. This will give great difficulty and probably be left in the jaw, the root breaking above the ball. Other roots may break in the socket; and while the practice is not correct, operators, who are not thoroughly experienced will do well to restrain from too strenuous efforts to get these roots.

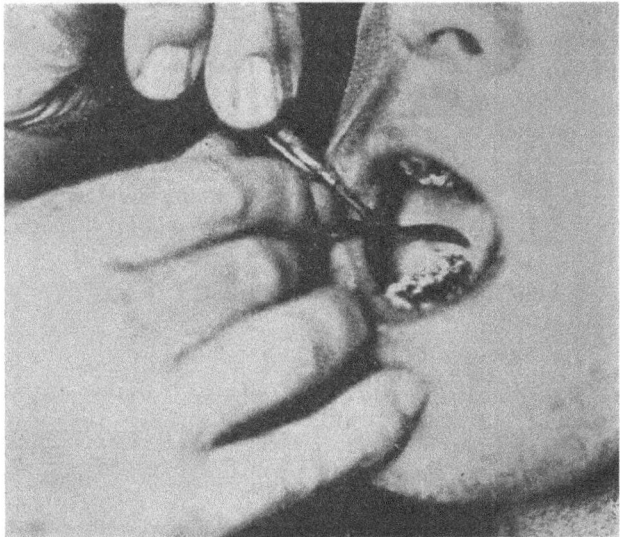

Fig. 45. — Lancing gums over erupting third molar, showing triangular incision, outer surface.

In the extraction of the upper molars and bicuspids the roots impinge closely upon and sometimes enter the cavity of the maxillary sinus. Faulty or forceful extraction is liable to bring out a large portion of the bone which forms the floor of this cavity, and serious complications result.

The extraction of the deciduous teeth or roots must be accompanied with caution, as to the distance the forcep beak is forced under the process since there is liability of injury to permanent teeth, which lie underneath.

In grasping a tooth through the alveolar process, in cases of roots deeply imbedded in the tissue, to force it from the socket by pressure on either side of the alveolar plate, application of too much force is liable to carry away a large quantity of the process. The reverse of this, the introduction of the beaks of the forceps, which are too thick, between the root and process is liable to sever or spread the process to the extent of fracture.

The opposite teeth are easily fractured by slipping forceps and a guard should be made by a finger of the opposite hand. There is danger of the tooth falling into the throat, after removal from the socket, in withdrawing it from the mouth, especially is this true of the wisdom teeth, if extracted with forceps which have too large a bow in the beaks.

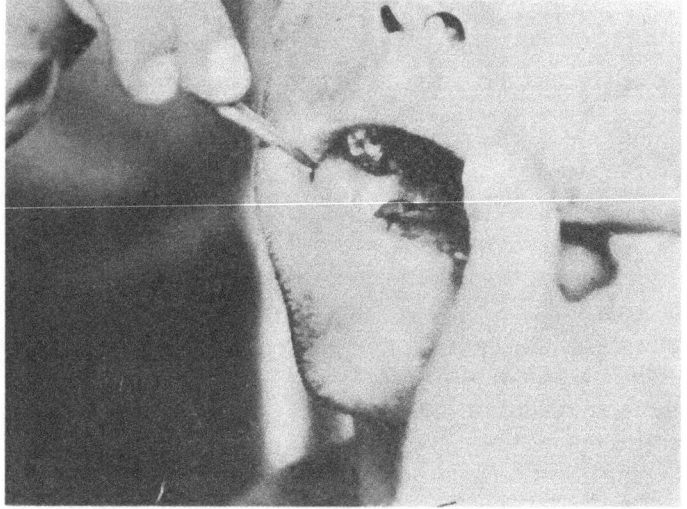

Fig. 46. — Lancing gums over erupting third molar, showing triangular incision, inner surface.

The *patient* should always be placed in such a position that the operator may have full view of the tooth, or that the fingers of the left hand may guard the beaks from the danger of including another tooth.

Precaution from infection during the operation should be taken. Large exposed wounds or sockets should be kept clean with a hot solution of one of the antiseptic mouth washes previously mentioned, until granulation begins and the socket closes. The treatment of infected sockets will be taken up later.

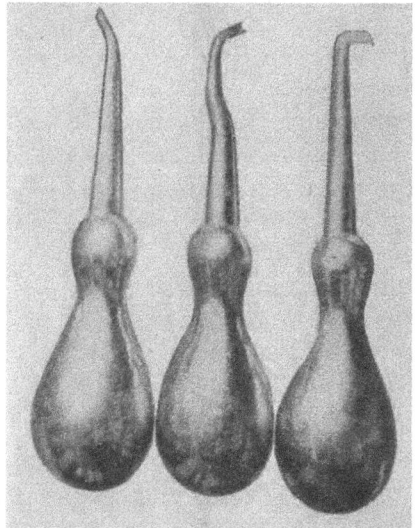

Fig. 47. — Elevators to be used in the extraction of roots.

The practice of lancing the gums, in extraction of teeth with crowns and a free gum margin, is not always advised; but with roots, it is seldom that the slitting of the gum is not necessary.

To lance this tissue use a sharp, straight or curved lancet; and free the tissue from the root on either side for the reception of the beaks of the forceps, or make a short incision on the inner and outer gum surface parallel to the root and through to the bony process.

In the lower wisdom teeth, if extraction is contemplated, or eruption to be aided, cross lancing is not advised, but a triangular piece of the gum should be removed. Make an incision from a high posterior point over the tooth to-ward the outer surface. Fig. 45 and then one on the inner as shown in Fig. 46 and then by a cross incision, remove the gum tissue thus severed. If this tooth is to be extracted it will be a simple matter to grasp the tooth with the forceps.

In preparing to extract a tooth, take the mouth mirror and with an explorer go all around the tooth and notice its attachment, its roots, and the angle as which it sets in the process. The writer then paints the tooth and surrounding tissue with tincture of iodine. Many times infection which lies in and around the tooth is carried down into the sockets. This procedure seems to prevent this, the iodine exerting the antiseptic action.

The *choice of the forceps* should be made with consideration of four points, viz., 1. The shape and the size of the beak should fit the tooth or root and not obstruct the view of the tooth. 2. The handles should fit the hand of the operator when the beaks are separated to the point necessary to grasp the tooth and the handles should be serrated to aid the grip so that the sensitiveness of the hand to resistance in extraction will not be destroyed. 3. They should be of proper material (good steel) and not bend or break under stress. 4. They should be cleaned and sterilized before using.

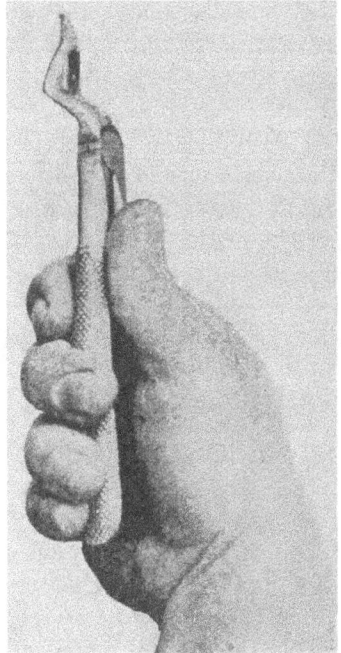

Fig. 48. — Position of hand and thumb gripping forceps for upper anterior teeth and roots.

The large number of forceps on the market represents many particular kinds devised by individuals and some of these cannot be used by most operators. Doubt is felt as to whether they can be used with success by the men who devised them.

The extraction of teeth by elevators is at times very satisfactory, it is a simple matter to place the beak down into the socket and by a prying movement force the root from the socket. The extraction of each individual tooth and its root will be taken up, in detail.

The Procedure of Extracting

The knack or art of extracting does not depend upon the strength of the operator, but lies in the sensitiveness of the hand to the giving away of attachment and the resistance of the tooth. This should guide the operator in applying force of withdrawal, as the teeth should be loosened before removal is begun.

The writer places the patient as low as possible in the dental chair and attempts to keep the head as near a line of his waist as possible. This will keep the elbow down and afford a sort of fulcrum. If the elbow is above the line of control of the shoulder muscles, difficulty will generally be experienced. The patient is tipped back for all of the upper teeth and sits upright for all of the lower. The protection of the lips must be made by the fingers of the left hand.

Extraction of the Upper Teeth

Examine all teeth surrounding with a mirror.

Central Incisors

One large, strong, round, conical root; select forceps shown in Fig. 48, or similar pair.

Take position as shown in Figs. 50 or 51.

Place inner beak of forceps well up on lingual surface at edge of enamel, genii)' close the forceps over the outer surface and with a rotary movement, force the beaks under the gums until they touch the alveolar process Fig 52.

Rotate and twist; using an "in-and-out" motion if resistance so demands; when loosened withdraw straight from the socket. Press alveolar walls together with the thumb and linger.

The extraction of the root of this tooth is practically the same procedure, except where it is broken off far under the process and it cannot be gripped with the forceps, then after lancing the gums parallel to the root, place the beaks of a root forceps as shown in Fig. 53 and pressure

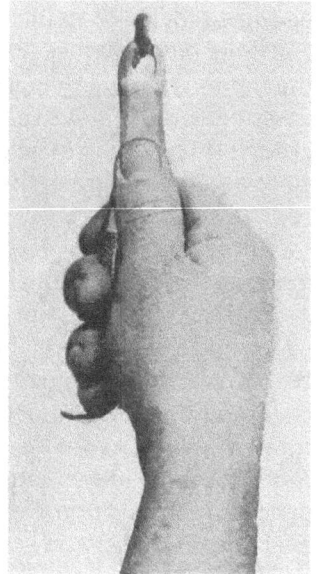

Fig. 49. — Position of hand gripping forceps, thumb placed between handles to prevent crushing tooth.

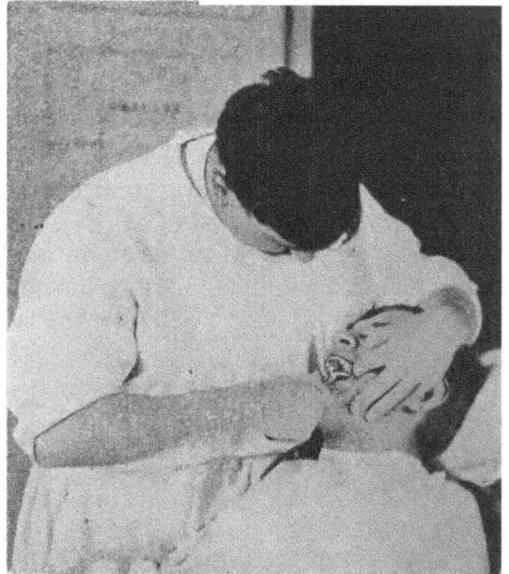

Fig. 50. — Position for operator. Extraction of teeth — upper left side of jaw.

will generally spring the tooth from the socket.

The Lateral Incisor

One small, flattened root, curved somewhat toward the canine.

Use same forceps as for central.

Take the same position.

Apply the forceps the same as with the central.

Place forceps on the tooth in the same manner.

Use an "in-and-out motion" and if resistance is felt, use a rotary movement. Any movement may be used which the operator feels, in his hand, is breaking the attachment.

Withdraw the tooth, when loosened, directly from the socket. Press alveolar walls, with the thumb and finger.

The extraction of the lateral root is practically the same as that of the central incisor.

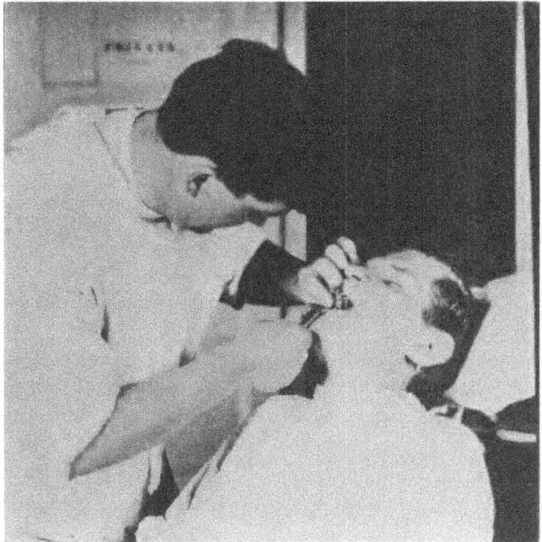

Fig. 51. — Position of operator. Extraction of teeth — upper right side of jaw.

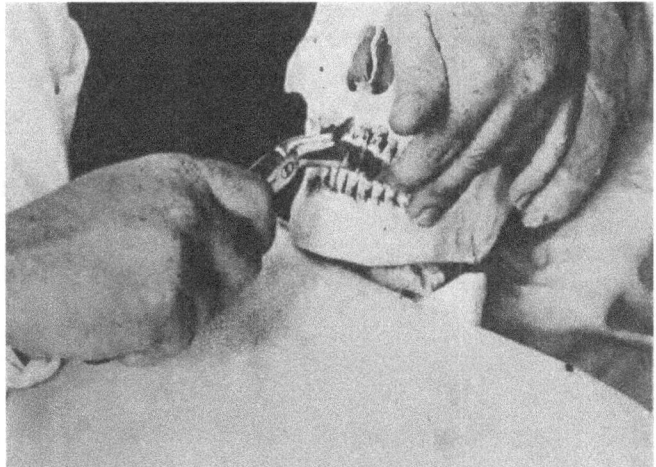

Fig. 52. — Extraction of upper incisor teeth.

The Cuspid or Canine
(Called the Eye Tooth)

One long, slightly flattened round root.

Sets in the jaw more firmly than any other tooth. Last to erupt, therefore frequently malposed and the root wedged between the lateral and bicuspid.

Roots project at times into the maxillary sinus.

Use forceps shown in Fig. 48 or one with a straight beak.

Apply forceps on the tooth in the same manner as shown in Fig. 54.

This tooth is at times twisted and pressure on the forceps should be applied "in and out," in a line of itsgreatest thickness, a rotating movement will be used to advantage and sometimes a backward motion. The sensitiveness of the hand will show the line of least resistance. When loosened it is usually easily removed. Press alveolar walls together with thumb and finger.

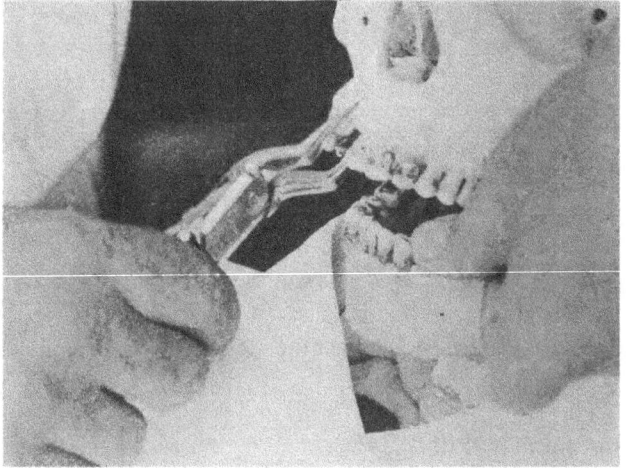

Fig. 53. — The extraction of the upper anterior roots. Forceps in position to compress or cut through the alveolar process.

The extraction of the root is practically the same as the tooth, except where it is broken under the process. In this case, lance the gum to the bone on the labial side, observe the direction of the root, and if wedged remove a small portion of the process with elevator No. 1, Fig. 47, place beak of forceps well up on the inner side and remove straight out from the labial process.

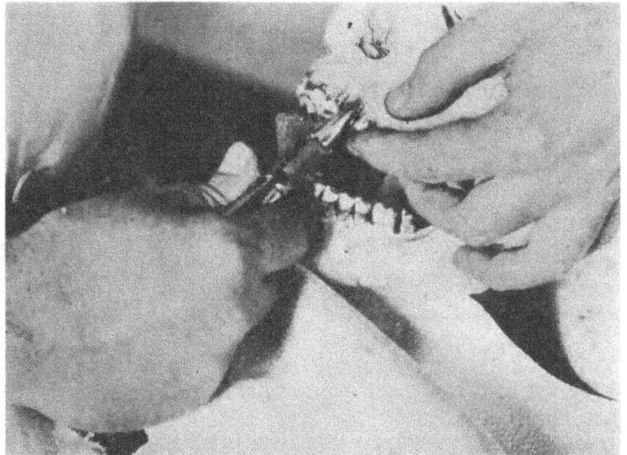

Fig. 54. — Forceps in position. Extraction upper cuspid.

First and Second Bicuspids

The first bicuspid: Usually two small, divergent roots which are generally round.

Use forceps shown in Fig. 55, and apply in same manner as incisors.

Take position as shown in Fig. 50 or 51.

Use an "in-and-out" motion. The tooth will loosen in many cases but not be easily removed because of the bony process within the bifurcation. Carrying the tooth outward will generally bring the tooth away, the outer alveolar process being thinner than the inner. In case difficulty occurs, these roots can be separated and removed with the root forceps, shown in Fig. 53.

The second bicuspid has a single slightly flattened root. Occasionally there are two.

The application of the forceps and extraction is practically the same as the first bicuspid.

The roots of these teeth will be removed with the forceps shown in Fig. 53. If one root of a double-rooted tooth remains, place one beak of the forceps in the socket and the other under the gums, and process. Its extraction will be simple.

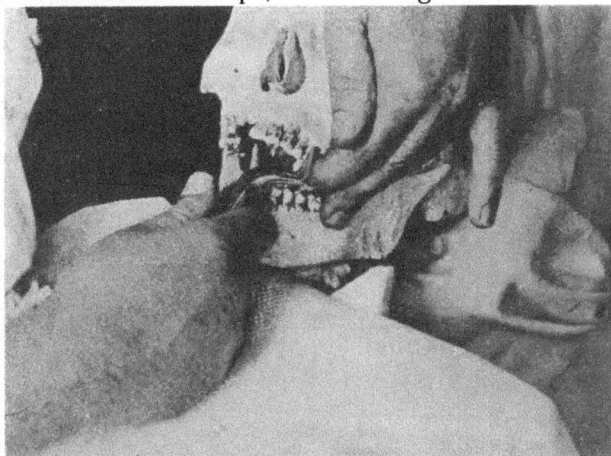

Fig. 55. — Extraction of upper left bicuspids, showing guard of finger behind forceps.

The First and Second Molars

These upper molars are very similar and the procedure in one the same as in the other, they both have three roots, one palatal (inside) and two buccal (outside). Consult Fig. 14. They vary in degrees of separation and there is no set rule for their extraction.

These teeth are the most commonly broken by inexperienced operators, by cutting the crowns with too much pressure on the forceps. Forceps Fig. 56 has grooves divided by a point on the outer beak, which fits between the buccal roots. A right and left pair of this forceps must be used.

Apply forceps well down under the gums, and with the thumb

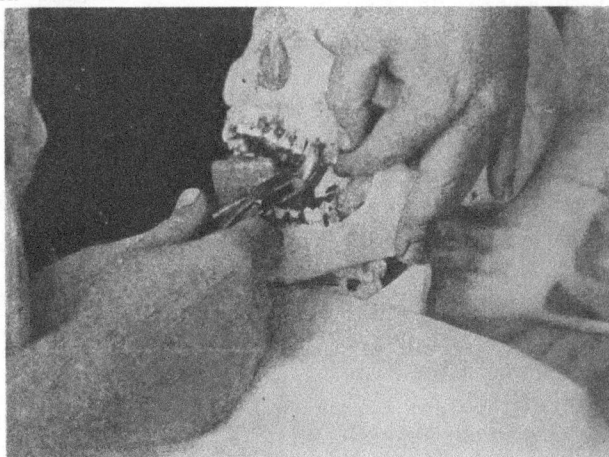

Fig. 56. — Extraction of upper left molars.

pressed between the handles to prevent too great a pressure on the beaks, force with an inward motion. This places the inner beak well up on the single

67

root and then force outward gripping tightly. When the beak is felt to go between the roots, proceed with a slow, steady, inward movement, the outer roots will give. The inner root will follow generally in the reverse outward motion.

Rocking the tooth will loosen the attachment. Rotalion is impossible.

Withdraw outward.

The roots of these teeth to be removed when the crown is missing should be taken one at a time. Use root forceps shown in Fig. 53. Take the anterior root first, with a direct in-and-out motion. The other buccal root, with rotary motion, and lastly the palatal root, the outer beak being placed in one of the empty sockets, apply pressure upward and then remove in the line of the direction of the root, outward and downward.

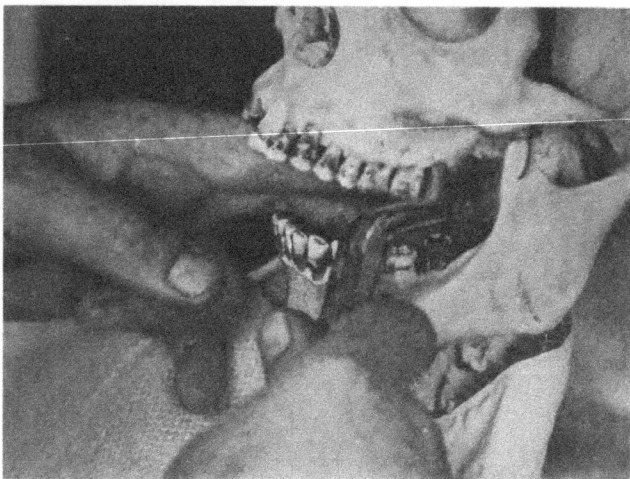

Fig. 57. — Extraction of upper left third molar wisdom tooth, showing fingers guarding against dropping the tooth down the patient's throat.

The Third Molar (Wisdom Tooth)

The number of roots varies from one to seven. The majority have one and three. The upper third molar is the easiest tooth extracted.

The bayonet-shaped forceps, Fig. 48, in the writer's experience is the

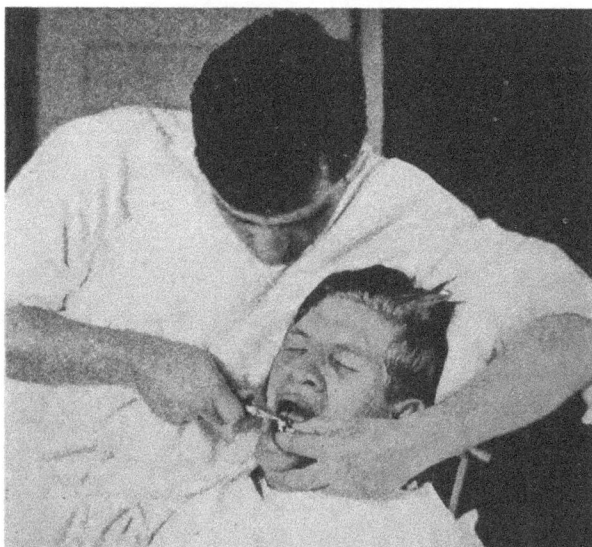

Fig. 58. — Position of operator. Extracting teeth, lower central incisors. Protection of lips with fingers of left hand.

best shape to be used, although the forceps shown in Fig. 57 is larger and heavier and in inexperienced hands may prove more satisfactory. Fake position as with other teeth on the proper side, Fig. 50 or Fig. 51. Place outer beak over the buccal surface of the tooth and bring inner beak to place, force the forceps up in the line which it now stands. Grip the tooth and turn upward and outward; an inward motion does no good until the tooth is loosened in the socket.

The fingers may be placed inside the mouth as shown in Fig. 57, just before removal to prevent the tooth from slipping through the forceps into the throat.

The inner alveolar plate is very thick and the outer one thin, so the in-and-out motion is not used.

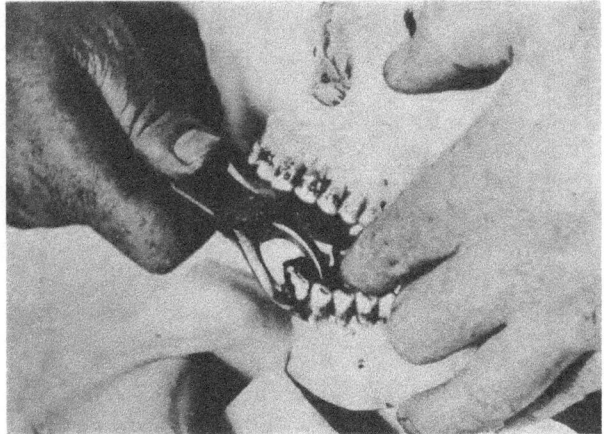

The Lower Teeth

Fig. 59. — Forceps in position. Extraction lower incisor.

The lower teeth are more difficult to extract than the upper ones because of the inability to see them as well.

The cheeks and the lips are more obstructive and the tongue, is generally in the way. Care must always be taken not to tear the gums or catch the tongue in the forceps.

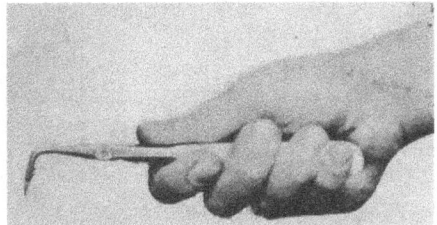

Fig. 60. — Position of hand and thumb gripping forceps for lower anterior teeth and lower roots.

The Central and Lateral Incisors and Canine

These teeth have all straight compressed roots except the cuspid which is sometimes wavy and rounded. Their extraction will be considered in one description.

Position as shown in fig. 58.

Carry the lips away with the left hand and apply the forceps as shown in Fig. 59, press firmly down under the gums and with an inward and outward motion rock the tooth and when loosened withdraw. Care must be taken in withdrawing these teeth, not to let the forceps strike the upper teeth when the tooth comes out.

The canine will give some trouble, as this root is much longer than the others and being rounded a rotary motion will be added to the above process.

The roots of these teeth will seldom be presented for extraction, neither will the teeth except when loosened by pyorrhea alveolaris.

The Lower First and Second Bicuspids

The roots of the first and second bicuspids are generally the same. The first, however, has two canals, but the roots are generally not separated.

They are compressed and round and slightly flattened.

The position will be taken as shown in Fig. 61 or 62.

The forceps may be used as shown in Fig. 58 or 64, and applied as shown in Fig. 64.

Press down well and rock the tooth with a direct inward and outward motion, until the tooth is loosened and then withdraw it. These teeth will generally give little trouble if the forceps are properly applied.

Press the alveolar process together with the finger and thumb.

Their roots are somewhat difficult to extract if broken off under the process.

Lance to the bone on either side and with the root forceps shown in Fig. 60, squeeze through the process and the tooth can be withdrawn.

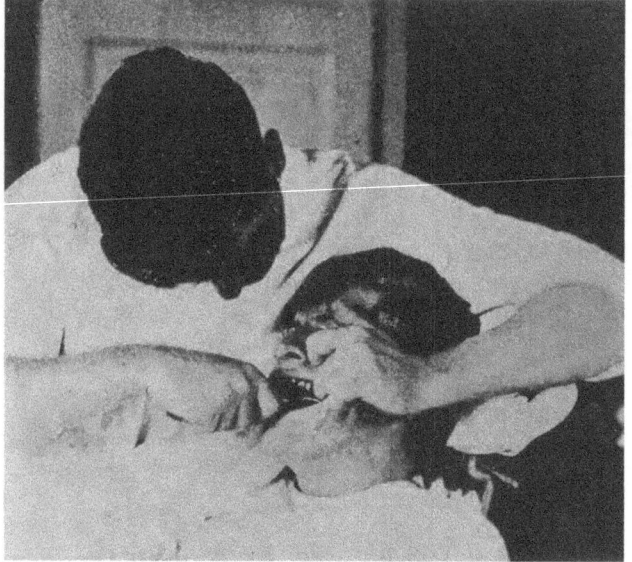

Fig. 61. — Position of operator. Extraction of teeth — lower left side of jaw.

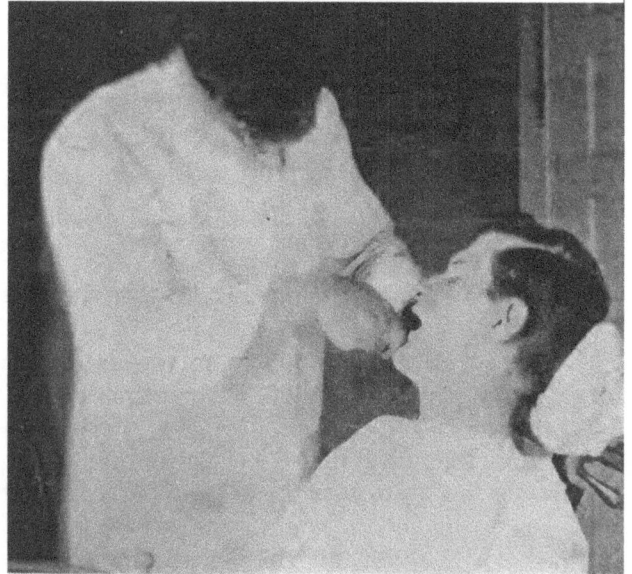

Fig. 62. — Position of operator. Extraction of teeth — lower right side.

70

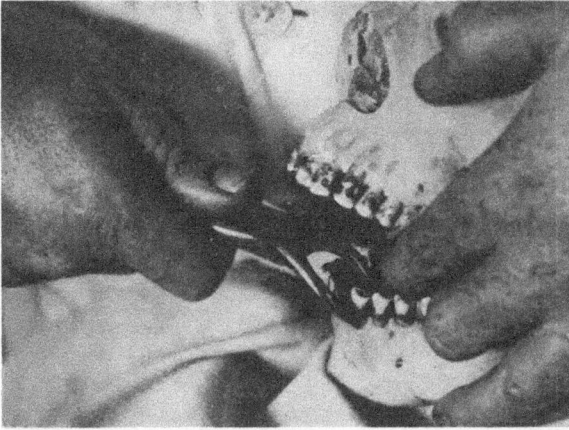

Fig. 63. — Forceps in position. Extraction lower cuspid.

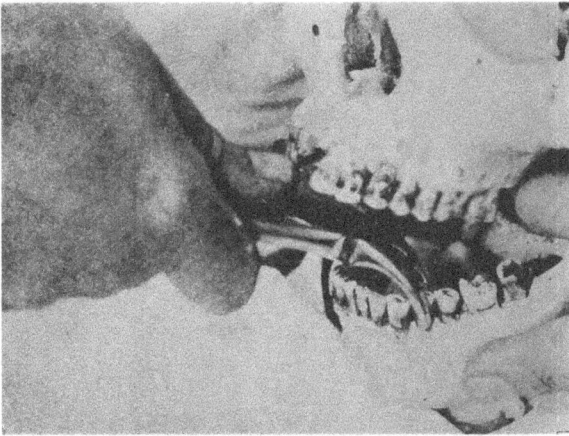

Fig. 64. — Extraction of lower left bicuspids.

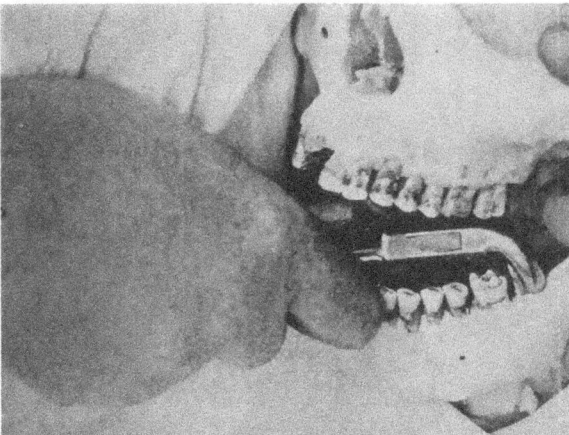

Fig. 65.— Extraction of the lower left first molar.

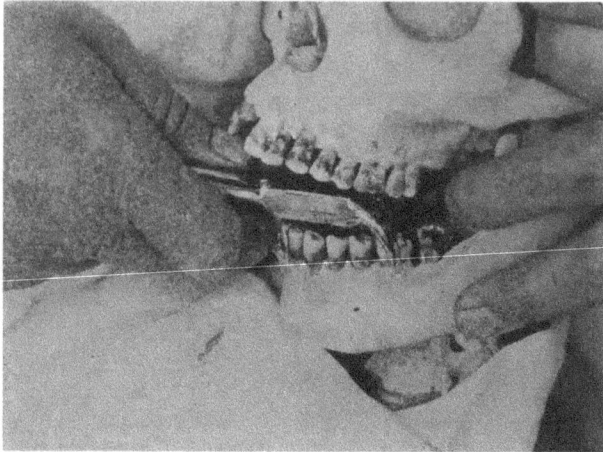

Fig. 66. — Extraction of lower molars with a hornbeak forceps.

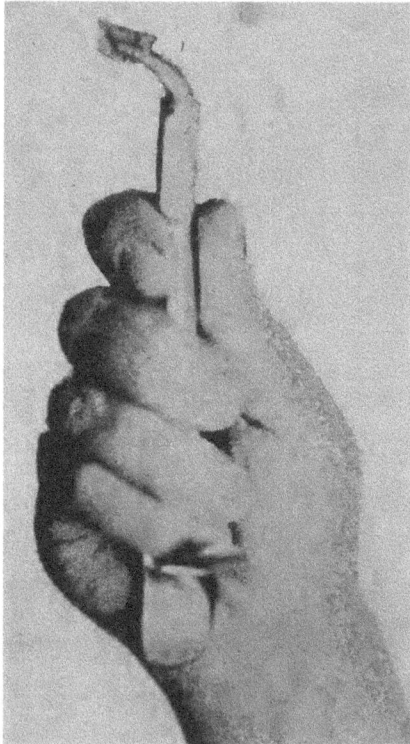

Fig. 67.— Position of hand, gripping hornbeak forceps for lower molar, side view of thumb between handles to prevent crushing.

The Lower First Molar

Two long roots, generally curved backward, slightly. Consult Fig. 14, Chapter V. One anterior and one posterior root, which are separated about the center of the tooth. Molar forceps are made with points and grooves on the beaks to fit in this space, between the roots, Fig. 65. Fig. 66 shows a "horn-beak" forceps in proper position, the points of the beaks here are received in the separation of the roots, Fig. 67.

The forceps are pressed well down until the beaks go home around the roots. The tooth is rocked in and out and will generally give way and then may be removed. Sometimes, however, it is necessary to keep up this motion while withdrawing from the socket.

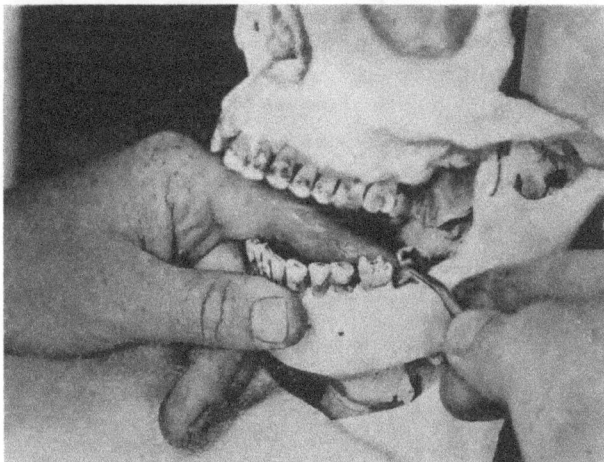

Fig. 68. — The elevator in position for the extraction of roots.

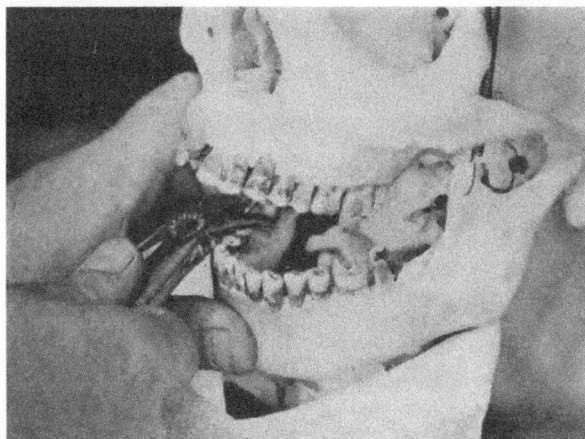

Fig. 69. — Extraction of lower right second molar.

The roots of this tooth are more prone to break than others and will be removed with the lower root forceps, Fig. 58. With only one root remaining in the socket the elevator as shown in Fig. 68 may be inserted in the empty socket and the root pried from its seat.

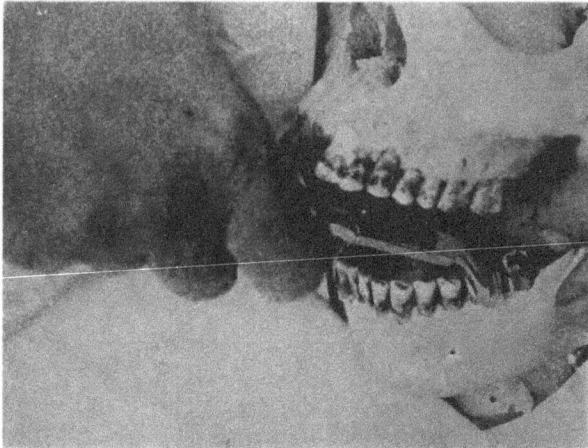

Fig. 70. — The extraction of the lower left second molar.

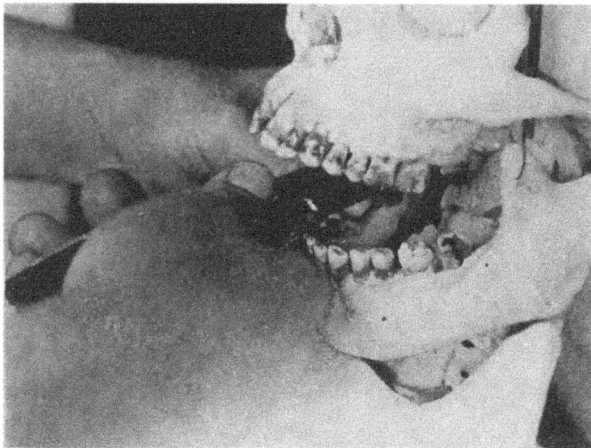

Fig. 71. — The extraction of lower third molars, wisdom teeth.

The Second Molar

Two roots, the same in the first molar, but not so diverging. Consult Fig. 14, Chapter Five. The same forceps used and the same procedure in the extracting as the first molar; using an in-and-out motion, and again being careful to have the beaks well down in the bifurcation of the roots. Figs. 69 and 70.

The Third Molar (Wisdom Tooth)

This tooth is the most difficult of all to extract because of its varying number of roots and its frequent malposition.

Take a position as shown in Fig. 61 or 62, right or left, select a forcep with a short thick beak or the lower root forceps, Fig. 58. Forceps shown in Fig. 69 can also be used to good advantage, except that there is a possibility of the tooth slipping out of the beaks into the throat.

Place the inner beak over the inside of the tooth and guided by the fingers of the left hand, the outer end is brought to place, Fig. 71.

The large thickness of bone on the outside of this tooth renders the outward motion useless. Turn the tooth directly inward, keeping a good pressure on the forceps.

This is just the opposite to the process necessary in the upper third molar.

These teeth are malposed, at times to such

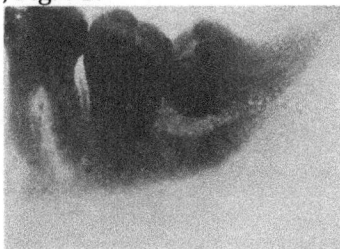

Fig. 72. — Impacted third molar. Radiograph. — *(Author's practice.)*

an extent that without an operation which first aid in extracting would justify, their extraction is impossible. Impactions often occur such as is shown in radiograph Fig. 72, and Fig. 73.

In Fig. 73 the tooth was erupting directly toward the outside. An inexperienced operator had failed in extraction of the second molar.

When impactions occur such as would necessitate an oral operation, the first aid or emergency might justify the extraction of the second molar, when in majority of cases the trouble will be ended.

The use of elevators, as shown in Fig. 68, may be very advantageous with these teeth.

An Improvised Dental Chair

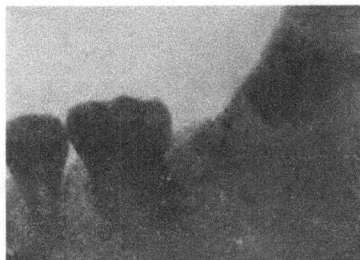

Fig. 73. — Impacted third molar, with fractured remains of lower second molar from faulty extraction by inexperienced operator. Radiograph. — *(Author's practice.)*

In the ordinary medical office, hospital or in the field, the question of a proper dental chair arises.

Figs. 74, 75 and 76 show the patient sealed in a common chair and the back of another resting against this, the left foot of the operator on the second chair, a head rest is made by the knee. Excellent results and control of the patient may be had in this manner.

The patient may push back and if he does this, the head will force the operator's knee down and press down on the chair at the back.

The head may be placed on any point of the operator's thigh to give a good view of the teeth to be extracted on either side of the mouth.

For the lower, Fig. 75, the head will be rested in the thigh and against the body of the operator.

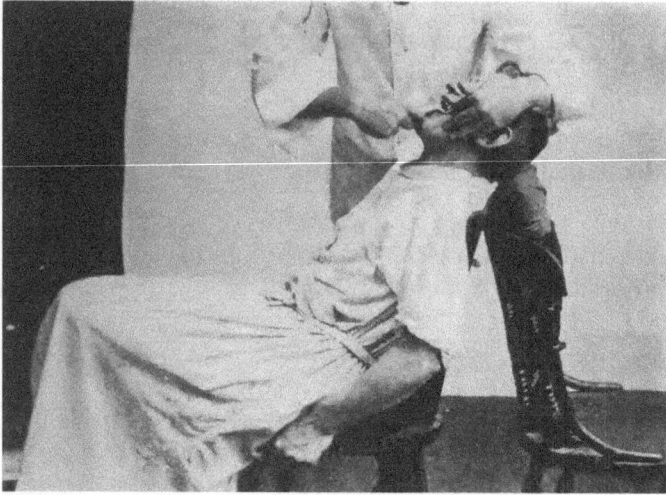

Fig. 74. — Position of patient and operator in improvised Dental Chair: Two common chairs placed back to back, patient's head on operator's knee. Extraction of upper teeth.

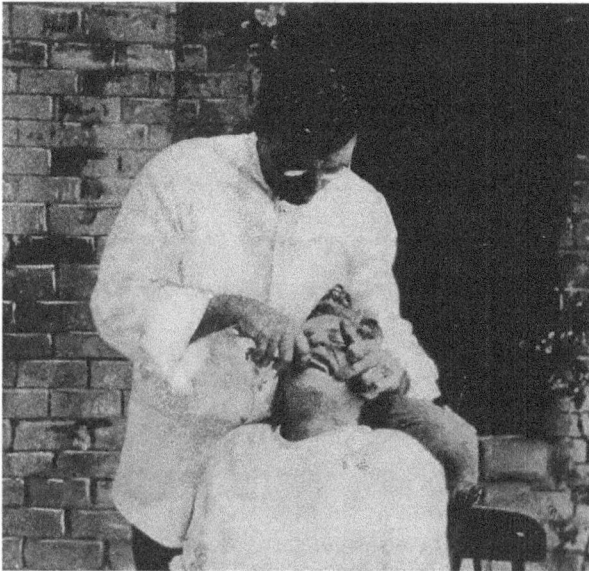

Fig. 75. — Improvised chair for extraction of the lower teeth, showing head resting on thigh and against body of operator.

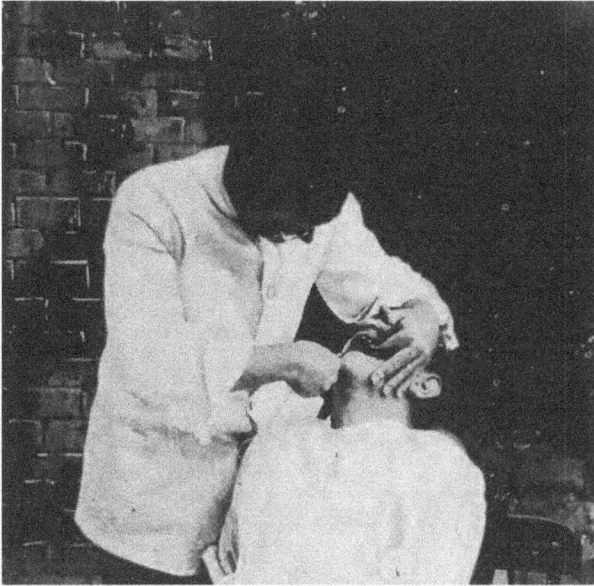

Fig. 76. — Extraction of upper teeth, left side. Same improvised chair.

Chapter Fourteen - Post-Operative Conditions

Pain after Extractions

Pain after extractions may be a result of injury to the peridental membrane or to the alveolar process; spreading or compressing its plates, or to the gum tissue.

The mouth being full of foul, septic matter, infection may later occur with resultant pain.

The mouth as stated before, should be syringed out with a good antiseptic wash and the instruments be absolutely sterile, then painting the parts with tincture of iodine will be considered a sufficient precaution.

Infection of sockets in many cases following the extraction of one or a number of teeth is unnecessary. If the proper precautions are taken it will occur only in a very small percentage of cases.

A record of five months of the writer's practice shows 1,161 teeth (including many badly necrosed roots) extracted with a result of four cases of infected sockets.

After the removal of the tooth and the compression of the alveolar process, the sockets will be washed out with a hot solution. No cotton or medicine of any kind should be placed in them.

If the gums are lacerated and the wound is gaping open, the cut or hanging tissue should be removed, with a small pair of curved scissors. Any points or jagged portions of the alveolar process should be broken down and smoothed over, with an elevator or a pair of forceps. Then paint' this part with tincture of iodine.

In case of pain, after this treatment, make a paste of iodoform, orthoform and campho-phenique and saturate a strip of gauze, fold this into the socket, leaving it for twenty-four hours.

A case dismissed may present in three or four days, with pain and infection in the socket. Wash out the mouth with a hot antiseptic and with a pair of tweezers and sterile cotton remove all the clot in the socket and flush out with a hot solution.

The writer paints this with a very small pledget of cotton saturated in tincture of iodine, and applies the above paste. The tincture of iodine does no special good in this case, where the paste is to be applied, except possibly to reduce the pain while inserting the gauze.

In nearly all cases of pain and infection, this paste will prove very efficient, the iodoform being antiseptic and the orthoform, a magic specific [1] for painful wounds, being a local anaesthetic, while the campho-phenique serves as a menstruum in mixing and appears to lessen the odor of the iodoform.

Hemorrhages after Extractions

Post-extraction hemorrhages may be very severe, even in the absence of hemophilia. These cases are not rare out are liable to be found at any time and must be dealt with wisely and promptly. All patients should be questioned as to liability of hemorrhage, or if "bleeders" (the common name for hemophiliacs) are in the family.

The death of a United States Senator, in recent years, was caused by hemorrhage from the extraction of a tooth and all known methods of treatment in this case were exhausted.

Hemorrhage from a socket may be capillary or arterial, and unless the patient is of a hemorrhagic diathesis, little difficulty will be experienced in stopping the bleeding.

Slight bleeding will yield sometimes to the holding of ice water over the socket. If no ice can be had a very hot solution will serve, used as hot as the patient can stand it.

The use of persulphate of iron should not be resorted to until all other remedies fail.

If the cold or hot water does not stop the flow, the paste of iodoform, orthoform and campho-phenique on a folded piece of gauze, packed tightly in the socket will answer in most cases. A gauze pack of tannic acid in glycerine will serve also, forced to the bottom of the socket. These packs will be observed daily and left until there is no danger of recurrence.

In hemophilia, the use of tampons and mechanical appliances will be necessary. The writer recommends the insertion of a gauze strip, longer than will be necessary, saturated with the paste of glycerite of tannin, folded upon itself to the bottom of the socket, when the gauze is flush with the gums, cut off the excess, fit a piece of cork over the socket, letting it extend down into the opening and trim it to the height of the teeth. Pressure is then made on this by a figure-of-eight ligature around the two teeth adjoining the socket, which serves to hold it in position. This cork may be held in place also, by the use of the Barton bandage, the former is preferable, when the teeth are present for attachment of the ligatures.

In extreme cases, the tooth antiseptically treated may be replaced in the socket.

The internal treatment should be conducted by the surgeon who will administer drugs which increase the coagulability of the blood. Those most commonly used are calcium chloride and calcium Lactate, 3-10 grains or 0.2 to 0.6-gm. doses.

Fainting

Patients may faint in the operations on the teeth or even before, from the sight of the instruments or from fear.

The condition is the result of the passing of the blood from the head, especially the brain, which becomes anemic. It is generally merely a physical problem to lower the head and let the blood run back. A patient who turns pale and blanches may have his head lowered between his knees for a few moments, which will revive him.

Dashing cold water in the face or the odor of ammonia will aid. In case these methods fail, from 10 to 20 drops of aromatic spirits of ammonia in water may be given, this being a cardiac and respiratory stimulant.

In extreme cases a pearl of amyl nitrite may be broken in a handkerchief and held close to the patient's nose.

[1] Buckley.

Chapter Fifteen - Diseases of the Maxillary Sinus-Antrum of Highmore

This chapter is intended for *Surgeons* and *Dental Surgeons* only.

The operations and care of the above conditions must be considered under emergency treatment, although not strictly first aid.

The surgeon or dental surgeon where the diagnosis of the condition is determined, cannot fail to see the necessity for emergency treatment. The methods of operation and treatment here described have given the writer and others such results that they are highly recommended.

Diseases of the maxillary sinus are much more common than is supposed "they are common among the lower class of society, or people who neglect their teeth." [1] There are various diseased conditions found affecting the sinus, among which are suppurative inflammation of purulent empyema, mucous engorgement, syphilitic ulceration, necrosis of the bony walls, tumors and dentigerous cysts, containing unerupted teeth, deciduous permanent or supernumerary.

This chapter will consider only the suppurative inflammation or purulent empyema, which has for its etiology, local conditions and diseases of the teeth, injurious catarrhal affections, foreign bodies, present in the cavity and dentigerous cysts.

All of the diseases of the teeth that have been taken up in this book which are located in the root canals, are etiological factors, especially those with putrescent pulps and acute and chronic abscesses. The roots of the superior teeth, as previously shown, the cuspids, bicuspids and molars, are separated from the cavity by a thin floor of bone. In the formation of abscesses, this tissue is easily destroyed and the drain of the pus is directly into the sinus.

Injuries, which fracture the bones of the face are prone to result in infection of the sinus, especially if the wound communicates with the mouth and gives access to the oral fluids. Other injuries spoken of as causes of empyema are the fracture of the process and the removal of portions of the floor in extraction of the teeth.

Among common causes are the catarrhal affections of the nasal tract resulting in the inflammation of its membrane which is continuous with the membrane lining the maxillary sinus.

Another cause is the presence of foreign bodies in the sinus, and in this class of causes dentigerous cysts are first to be considered. Nature tries to expel the teeth forcibly and they become sources of irritation and result in severe cases of pus formation. Other foreign bodies such as dental material, root-fillings, etc., may be forced through the root into this cavity. Insects may be taken in through the nose and find their way into this sinus.

The symptoms of suppuration of the sinus are pain, dull and deep-seated, which later becomes intense and extends over the whole side of the head and face. The walls of the Antrum of Highmore become thin and Marshall states that under pressure they give forth a crackling sound like that of the crushing of an egg shell.

The orbit forming the roof of the sinus, suppuration exerts its pressure on this and at times forces the eyeball to a marked protrusion and causes paralysis of the optic nerve from this force.

If the discharge of pus is directed into the nose, the odor of the breath is very offensive. The condition is clearly one demanding prompt and decisive action.

The diagnosis is at times somewhat difficult. Theuse of a light shadowing through the sinus, the soreness, pain and swelling on the side of the face affected. In unilateral or both, if bi-lateral, the presence of pus escaping through the nose, when the head is held down and quickly thrown back and to the opposite side, the soreness of the teeth, the crepitus of the thinner part and the X-ray for foreign bodies are the means of diagnosis. The radiograph is the most satisfactory method of locating foreign bodies and determining the condition.

Treatment

In every disease, the removal of the cause is the first thing to be considered, so with the maxillary sinus affections, but when the cavity is full of pus, it demands primarily, opening and drainage.

A local anaesthetic or Nitrous Oxide and Oxygen or other general anaesthetic may be used. A 2 per cent, solution of eucaine or cocaine as a local anaesthetic is used with success, but novocaine is preferable to either of these and all other local anaesthetics.

There are many methods of operating for this condition. Some operators extract the first molar or bicuspid tooth and

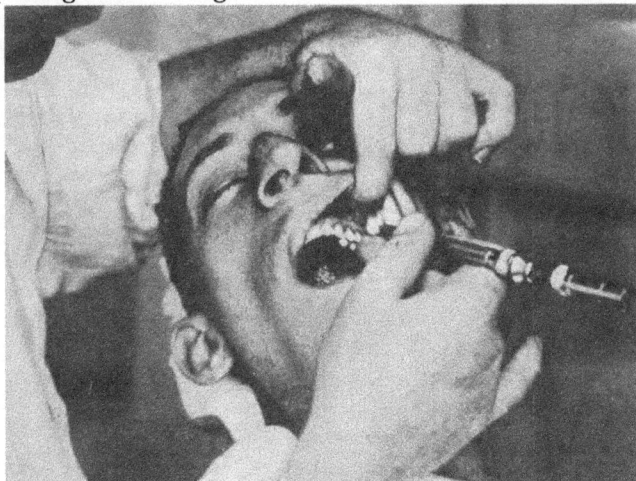

Fig. 77. — Empyema of the Antrum of Highmore, position showing method of opening with drill, with gutta-percha guard, between the roots of the second bicuspid and the buccal root of the first molar.

make an entrance into the sinus, through the sockets of these with a trephine or engine drill. Marshall has devised an excellent trocar and canula for this operation and in this method of entrance it is very desirable.

The writer recommends the method shown in Fig. 77. A root reamer burr is selected for the dental engine. The distance determined that the drill should enter and a gutta-percha ball placed on the burr at this point, to prevent its slipping and puncturing the floor of the orbit. Make an incision well up over the side of the roots of the second bicuspid and first molar teeth; insert the drill between the roots. An opening as large as an ordinary lead pencil will suffice for suppuration, unless the removal of foreign matter requires a larger one. This is the best place in the mouth to open into the antrum because it is a dependent portion and is better than going through a tooth socket because the food and oral secretions do not have access; since the cheek covers the wound. Where the dental engine is not available or desired, the chisel and hammer may be nicely used, the opening being made large

81

enough to admit exploration with the fingers if desired to remove foreign bodies.

E. J. Craig of Kansas City has a method of making a drain as follows: Take a silver wire, 20 gauge, wind it over a handle slightly smaller than the opening, to make a close coil about 1 inch in length; this may be bent in any direction. Insert it in the opening and keep it there for one or two days. Flatten the outer end so that it will not irritate the buccal tissue. This drain will not work through into the antrum as many drains are liable to do and it affords entrance for the syringe tip. The opening will not close after its removal if left for two or three days.

The cavity should be syringed out with a normal salt solution, 100° temperature from a Moffat syringe, or a fountain syringe, with a glass nozzle made to fit the case, the bag containing the water held not higher than the patient's head, in the first few sittings.

The use of 10 per cent, argyrol solution is an excellent remedy after the drain has been perfected through the nose. Harlan recommends in chronic cases, after irrigating as long as deemed necessary, flooding the cavity with a 2 per cent, silver nitrate solution, which makes a profound impression on the tissues and further treatment is unnecessary.

In chronic cases which have large openings, from an operation to remove foreign matter, the bismuth paste given in a previous chapter is injected by some operators with great success. The cavity after operation is packed with this paste on gauze, continuing the washing with the warm saline solution for time desired. An operation for a typical case of dentigerous cyst was performed at a convention of the New York State Dental Society, by Dr. Henry Sage Dunning, of New York, Dr. Dunning has very kindly furnished the following description of same with use of plates.

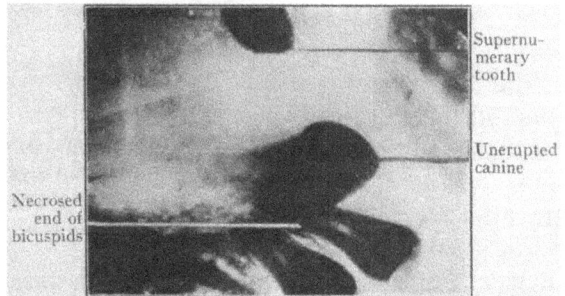

Fig. 78. — **Dentigerous cyst in the maxillary sinus. Radiograph. — (Dr. Dunning's practice.) Case cited.**

"*Patient,* young Swede, seventeen years old, came to clinic complaining of swollen face, upper right side and slight pain. Patient said that the face had been swollen for about eight to ten months. Sometimes swelling would increase and become hard and then would get smaller or go down and patient thinks he would at this time notice a discharge in the mouth.

Examination. — Face, swelling of face marked, extending from infraorbital region to alveolar process and from ala of nose to zygomatic arch, the entire wall of antrum was ballooned anteriorly about ½ to ¾ of an inch. Bony wall of antrum greatly thinned out and a distinct egg-shell crackle noted. Somewhat tender, above area somewhat red and slightly warmer than on other side. Fig. 78.

Mouth, central lateral, first bicuspid, second bicuspid, first and second molar in position, and in good condition. Third molar erupting, canine missing, and space of ½ inch between lateral and first bicuspid. Marked swelling over alveolar ridge, extending from canine fossae to second molar region. This swelling was oval in shape and was about the size of a pigeon egg. External plate was thin and egg-shell crackle noted as on face. Small sinus noticed just over the lateral and probe could be passed along neck of this tooth into its alveolus, up into large cavity for a distance of about 1 inch. X-ray showed non-erupted permanent canine just over lateral root, and above this there was shown another tooth, which looked like a supernumerary tooth. Large cavity shown by X-ray to involve antrum, but unable to tell by film to what extent. Roots of the two bicuspids somewhat absorbed and extending into the cyst cavity.

Diagnosis. — A true dentigerous cyst, containing two teeth. Nose examined, negative; ear examined, negative.

Operation performed before the members of the New York State Dental Convention at Albany, New York. Patient given 1/6 grain morphine by hypodermic to quiet him and to relieve from post-operative pain. Cyst area painted with ½ strength iodine. One per cent, novocaine injected into swelling of alveolar border, deeply into periosteum and bone. An incision was then made along swelling, extending from lateral to second molar. Soft tissues laid back and bone exposed. Anterior wall of antrum found to be very thin; with chisel and mallet broke through thin external alveolar

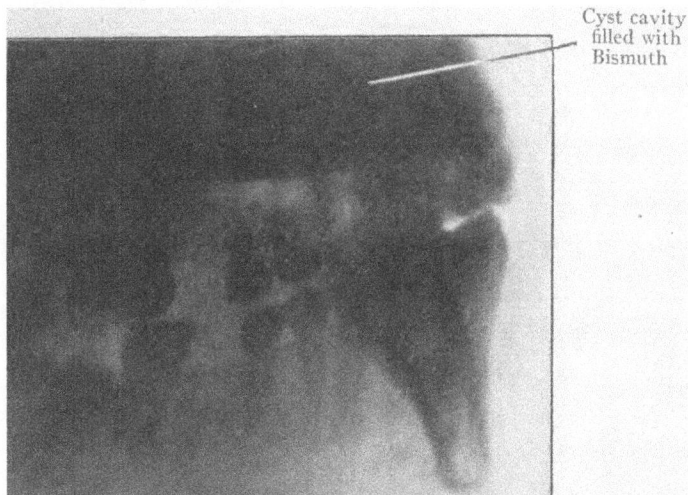

Cyst cavity filled with Bismuth

Fig. 79. — After operation-cavity filled with bismuth paste.

plate and found large cavity full of thick yellow pus, containing white flakes. Enlarged cavity quickly and entire wall of antrum found to be thin, soft and necrotic in places. With rongeur forceps removed large area of diseased anterior wall and made opening into the antrum, that would allow passage of ends of four fingers of hand. Excavated about 1¼ ounces of thick pus, irrigated the cavity with warm saline solution and for the first time obtained good view of the cavity. Cavity extended from floor to alveolar ridge of orbit, from second molar to lateral and upward to floor of nose. Cavity lined with smooth thin membrane or sac, which was partly removed by the operator. Cavity curetted and two teeth, a temporary canine and permanent canine dislodged from bony wall. Rough edges of thin bone surrounding opening into cavity smoothed off and cavity packed with bismuth paste and gauze. This cyst cavity was found to connect directly with the nose. The membrane lining the bone cavity seemed to wall off nose at middle meatus, the natural communication of the nose and antrum. A puncture through the nose, into the cavity was performed to establish better drainage.

Treatment. — Cavity has been packed with bismuth paste gauze and irrigated with warm saline solution about three times a week for the last three months. Opening has closed in considerable but cyst cavity about the same size. Tissues are clean and healthy.

Prognosis. — Opening into cyst cavity and antrum will continue to fill in, but will never completely close. No danger of recurrence, as lining of membrane of cyst has been removed and source of irritation, the teeth, has been removed. Fig. 79.

[1] Marshall.

Authors and Books Consulted

Abbott: "Principles of Bacteriology."

Allen: "Vaccine Therapy and Opsonic Treatment.", "American Text-book of Operative Dentistry."

Black: "Dental Anatomy."

Bodecker: "Anatomy and Pathology of the Teeth."

Broomell: "Anatomy and Histology of the Mouth and Teeth."

Buckley: "Modern Dental Materia Medica, Pharmacology and Therapeutics."

Burchard: "Dental Pathology, Therapeutics and Pharmacology."

Burchard and Inglis: "Dental Pathology and Therapeutics."

Burr, Aaron: "Dental Cosmos."

Cryer: "Internal Anatomy of the Face."

Da Costa: "Gray's Anatomy.", "Dental Cosmos."

Gorgas: "Dental Medicine."

Harlan: "Lectures."

Hunter: "Oral Sepsis." "Items of Interest."

Jackson: "Orthodontia."

Johnson: "Principles and Practice of Filling Teeth."

Keyes: "Syphilis."

Longmore: "Gunshot Wounds."

Marshall: "Injuries and Surgical Diseases of the Face, Mouth and Jaws."

Miller: "Micro-organisms of the Human Mouth."

Ottolengui: "Methods of Filling Teeth."

Prinz: "Dental Materia Medica and Therapeutics."

Stimson: "Fractures and Dislocations."

Talbot: "Interstitial Gingivitis."

Tomes: "Dental Surgery."

Wallis: "Atlas of Dental Extractions."

Zeigler: "Pathology."

www.ingramcontent.com/pod-product-compliance
Lightning Source LLC
Chambersburg PA
CBHW051849040426
42447CB00006B/764